Exam 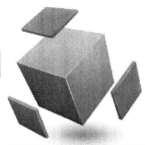 Facts

OCCUPATIONAL THERAPIST ASSISTANT

COTA

Certified Occupational Therapist Assistant Exam

Kori Callahan

Study Guide

Certified Occupational Therapist Assistant
COTA

EXAM FACTS

BY KORI CALLAHAN

FIRST EDITION

© EXAM FACTS

HTTP:\\WWW.EXAMFACTS.COM

U.S.A.

Table of Content

COTA – Certified Occupational Therapist Exam 1

Welcome 1

About The Author...2

Why Exam Facts?...2

Exam Information..3

Just the Facts...4

OT Review 4

Vision and Cognition..12

Allen Cognitive Levels 16

OT Terms 18

Splinting and Diagnoses......................................23

Pediatric Milestones 27

Pediatrics UE development 30

MET Levels...35

Wheelchair Measurements...................................39

Rancho Levels..43

MMT and Range of Motion 45

Spinal Cord Levels & Injury Concepts 47

SCI Therapeutic Intervention...............................55

Rood Facilitation Techniques 65

PNF (Proprioceptive Neuromuscular Facilitation) 68

Glascow Coma Scale 70

Pre-Writing Skills 70

Erik Erikson Stages of Development 71

Hip Fractures & Replacements.............................73

Assessments 74

COPM (Canadian Occupational Performance
Measure) 76

GENERAL OT 77

Arthritis 80

Psychotropic Medications....................................81

OT discipline and OTA/COTA info........................85

MISC FACTS..87

OT HISTORY..91

FRAMEWORKS 102

FIELD WORK 104

Abbreviations 114

    Patient Safety Abbreviations 139

COTA – Certified Occupational Therapist Exam

PASS THE COTA – CERTIFIED OCCUPATIONAL THERAPIST ASSISTANT EXAM BY USING EXAM FACTS "JUST THE FACTS" STUDY GUIDE.

The NBCOT (National Board of Certified Occupational Therapists) COTA examination is for any person who wants to be certified as an Occupational Therapist Assistant. Most, if not all states require a person to be certified by this examination to perform therapy.

Welcome

Thank you for choosing Exam Facts COTA Study Guide, First Edition. This book is part of a family of premium-quality Exam Facts books, all of which are written by outstanding authors who combine teaching experience with real life working experience.

Our goal is to bring you the best books available to help you succeed. I hope you see all that reflected in these pages. We would be very interested to hear your comments and get your input on how we can improve our products. Feel free to let me know what you think about this book or any other Exam Facts book by sending us an email at support@examfacts.com. If you think you've found a technical error in this book, please let us know and we will definitely research and correct it. Your response is critical to our efforts at here at Exam Facts.

1

Thank you,
Colton McGovney,
Chief Editor at Exam Facts.

About The Author

Kori Callahan was a former college teacher who shifted her focus to Occupational Therapy. She focused long nights going to school to become an Occupational Therapist Assistant. She then became a roving OTA instructor, who has taught Occupational Therapy in over 14 countries. This was on top of being married, running the household and raising two boys Kori is committed to provide readers the knowledge for you to be successful. With this edition, future financial candidates can rest assured that they will be receiving the latest study material available to advance their career.

Acknowledgement

Thank you to the many students who helped with our books. Your input is was critical in what we write.

Why Exam Facts?

We create study guides that are compiled facts that you need to know. No fluff, no long stories that can be distracting to what you really need to learn and remember. Some of our guides have questions filtered in but we try to give you facts, straight to the point so you remember and use that information in your deciphering and understanding of the test questions.

Exam Facts gets some of the best experts in each field to compile and write what is needed for you to be successful. We also get input from you, the test taker on what you'd like to see or if all possible, what we have missed.

We also strive to keep the price as low as possible, sometimes even a hundred dollars cheaper than other guides on the market.

Exam Information

COTA / Certified Occupational Therapist Assistant Examination

Exam Info:

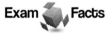

www.examfacts.com

TIME LIMIT:	4 hours
COST:	$500 US Online / $540 Paper Application as of August 2012. Note that this is the examination enrollment fee ONLY--other fees may also apply. Please visit the http://www.nbcot.org for more information.
NUMBER OF QUESTIONS:	200
PASSING SCORE:	Test is Scored on a rating scale (200-600)
FORMAT:	Multiple Choice
PREREQUISITES:	no
EXAM DATE(S):	See http://www.NBCOT.org
EXAM LOCATIONS:	See http://www.NBCOT.org
OFFICIAL EXAM WEBSITE:	http://www.nbcot.org

OT Review

Define briefly Tardive Dyskinesia
The involuntary rolling of the tongue and twitching of the face or trunk or limbs

Define briefly Akathisia
The inability to remain calm, still, and free of anxiety

Define briefly Myasthenia Gravis

A chronic progressive disease characterized by chronic fatigue
and muscular weakness, especially in the neck and face

Define briefly Guillan Barre
Symptoms include muscle weakness, mild distal sensory loss
and complaints of painful extremities

Define briefly Echopraxia
Repetitive imitation of another person's movements

Define briefly Ideational Apraxia
Uses objects incorrectly (ex: uses toothbrush to brush hair)

What is the Cognitive Performance Test?
Based on Allen's Cognitive Levels it is an assessment of 6 ADL
tasks that require cognitive skills

What is the Barthel Index?
A measurement of a person's independence in BADLs before
and after intervention and the level of personal care needed for
the individual

What is the Dynamic Interactional Approach
It emphasizes transfer of learning and varying treatment
environments

What is LOTCA (cognitive assessment)?
Often used for stroke, TBI and tumors, it measures basic
cognitive functions for managing everyday tasks

What are the AMPS (assessment of motor and process skills)
Determines functional competence in 2/3 familiar and chosen BADL/IADL tasks

What are Brunnstrom's levels of motor recovery?
Stage 1
The limbs (and trunk) are flaccid and the nervous system is in a state of inhibition. Muscle stretch reflexes (i.e., biceps, pronator, pectoralis major, triceps, quadriceps and tendon Achilles) are absent or hypoactive, the limbs will feel heavy and does not respond to facilitation. During the transition from Stage 1 to 2, tone increases. This increase in tone with the onset of hyperactive muscle stretch reflexes is obvious before active movement can be facilitated.
Stage 2
Active movement can be facilitated or occurs spontaneously as an associated reaction. Arm movement may result from facilitation of the tonic neck reflexes. Resistance given to the contralateral limb may also produce movement through facilitation of an associated reaction. Movement can be in any range. *For scoring purposes, do not consider an increase in tone alone to qualify as movement.* Movement results from the facilitation of spinal reflexes (e.g., input via cutaneous or proprioceptive receptors), brainstem (or tonic neck) reflexes (input via proprioceptive vestibular receptors or receptors in the neck), or associated reactions (irradiation from antagonists, synergists or muscles from the opposite side of the body).
Stage 3
Active voluntary movement occurs without facilitation, but is only in the stereotyped synergistic patterns.
Stage 4
Synergy patterns and simple movements out of synergy are possible at Stage 4.
Stage 5
Full range synergy movements and complex combinations of synergies are possible. Ankle eversion, hip abduction with internal rotation, and finger and thumb extension are

movements, which are not part of either the flexion or extension synergies.
Stage 6

Muscle movements are different from normal only when the nervous system is stressed. Requesting more complex or faster movement that will normally be needed in daily activities tests this.
Stage 7
There is no evidence of functional impairment. Activities and skill are at a pre-stroke level. There is a "normal" sensory-perceptual-motor system. Arms and legs do not feel heavier than the contralateral side nor do they fatigue more rapidly.

Define firm pressure and resistance
Less threatening than light touch

Define linear movement
Less threatening than angular movement

Define slow movement
Less threatening than rapid movement

What does OBRA (omnibus budget reconciliation act) state?
It mandates that restraints can't be used without proper justification, agreement, and documentation

What are door swing measurements for each of the following?
18 inches for walker
26 inches for Wheelchair

What are the ADA requirements for house?
32 inches= doorway
36 inches= hallway
31 inches high= countertops

What are the ramp requirements?
for every 1 foot of rise = 1 foot of ramp

What are Reisburgs stages of dementia?
1. No signs
2. Person complains of forgetting normal age related information
3. Beginning signs
4. IADL deficits
5. Can't function independently
6. ADL completed only with cues
7. Bedbound

What is astereognosis?
The inability to identify objects through touch

What is tangentially?
A change of focus to a loosely associated topic

What is circumstantiality?
Speech that is delayed in reaching the point of conversation

What is Rett Syndrome?

Progressive disorder that affects cognitive, motor, social, and language
Developmental reversals

What is seen with a Right CVA?
Poor judgment and safety difficulties

What is seen with a Left CVA?
Slow and cautious behavior, fearfulness and hesitancy

What are characteristics of the Symmetric tonic neck reflex?
Onset: 4-6 months
Stimulus: place infant in the crawling position and extend the head
Response: Flexion of the hips and knees
*Breaks up total extensor posture

What are characteristics of the Landau reflex?
Onset: 3-4 months
Stimulus: hold infant in horizontal prone suspension
Response: Complete extension of the head, trunk, and extremities
*Breaks up flexor dominance

What are the characteristics of the Labyrinthine/optical (head) righting reflex?
Onset: birth-2 months
Stimulus: hold infant suspended vertically and tilt slowly to the side, forward, and backward
Response: Upright positioning of the head
*Orients head in space/maintains face vertical

What are the characteristics of the Moro reflex?
Onset: 28 weeks gestation
Stimulus: rapidly drop infant's head backward
Response: First phase=arm extension; Second phase=arm
flexion and adduction
*protective response

What are the characteristics of the Galant reflex?
Onset: 32 weeks gestation
Stimulus: hold infant in prone suspension, gently scratch or tap
alongside the spine with finger, from shoulders to buttocks
Response: lateral trunk flexion and wrinkling of the skin on the
stimulated side
*facilitates trunk stabilization

What is Skier's Thumb (Gamekeeper's Thumb)?
Rupture of the ulnar collateral ligament of the MCP joint of the
thumb

What is the Kleinert protocol for flexor tendon repair?
Active extension of digit with passive flexion by using rubber
band traction
0-4 weeks: dorsal block splint. Passive flexion and active
extension within the splint
4-6 weeks: Wristlet. Place and hold exercises
6-8 weeks: AROM
8-12 weeks: Strengthening

What is the Duran protocol for flexor tendon repair?
Passive flexion and extension of digit
0-4 weeks: dorsal block splint. Passive flexion of joints.
4-6 weeks: active flexion and extension within the splint
6-8 weeks: tendon gliding
8-12 weeks strengthening

What is Pronator Teres Syndrome?
Medial nerve compression between two heads of pronator
Teres

What does the Supraspinatus do?
abduction and flexion

What do the Infraspinatus and Teres Minor do?
external rotation

What does the subscapularis do?
internal rotation

What is the Anti-deformity positions following burn injury?
Neck: neutral to slight extension
Axilla: (airplane splint) shoulder abduction 90 degrees and
external rotation
Elbow: extension
Forearm: neutral to supination
Wrist: 30-45 degree extension
Hand: MCPs 70 degree flexed, IP extended, thumb abducted

What are the classifications of heart disease?
1: No limits to activity
2: Slight activity limit, ordinary activity results in fatigue, pain,
dyspnea, palpitations
3. Marked limitations
4: Inability to carry out physical activity without discomfort

What is a typical adult heart rate?

60-80 bpm

Vision and Cognition

What is Myopia?
nearsightedness

What is Hyperopia?
farsightedness

What is Retinitis Pigmentosa?
decreased visual acuity, photophobia, constriction of visual field, night blindness

What is Glaucoma?
severe redness, pain in the eye, headache & nausea

What is Chronic Open Angle Glaucoma?
decreased visual acuity & peripheral fields, photophobia, no pain

What is Age-related Macular Degeneration?
central vision of macula is affected, causing scotomas (scarred areas), reduced contrast sensitivity

What are Cataracts?
cloudiness of the lens of the eye, decreased acuity, progressively blurred vision, both central and peripheral, glare sensitivity, near vision better than distant usually

What is Retinopathy?
decreased visual acuity, scarring, retinal detachment causing possible field loss or blindness

What is Albinism (related to vision)?
total or partial loss of pigment, decreased acuity, nystagmus, high refractive error, astigmatism

What is Diabetic Retinopathy?
Swiss cheese effect, spotted areas of vision, fluctuates based on glucose levels, decreased visual acuity, contrast sensitivity, color vision, night vision, temporary diplopia

How would a therapist determine possible visual acuity deficits?
Basic Observation: Client wanting more light, blurry or fuzzy when reading, tries bringing print into focus, changes head position often, unable to stay on line when writing

ADL Function: issues with reading, writing, fine motor coordination, socialization & communication with others, cooking, accessing phone for emergencies, driving

What are interventions for visual acuity deficits?
Intervention: community resources, larger print, lighting, magnification

How would a therapist determine Peripheral Visual Deficits?
Basic Observation: omits letters or words, loses place when reading, watches feet when walking, knocks into things, has poor eye contact, has a hard time navigating

ADL Function: frequently misses words, may shuffle feet walking, bumps & trips into things, locating friends or items is difficult

What are interventions for peripheral visual deficits?
Intervention: community resources, large print, increase lighting in rooms, control glare, yellow & amber sunglasses may help, scanning training, safety adaptations

How would a therapist determine Contrast Sensitivity Deficits?
Basic Observation: Difficulty-recognizing faces, trimming fingernails, distinguishing colors, stumbles frequently

ADL Function: reading, writing and fine motor tasks of difficulty contrasting print, cutting foods, disorganized space

What are interventions for Contrast Sensitivity Deficits?
Intervention: change color to increase contrast, decrease patterns, and reduce clutter, environmental adaptations

How would a therapist determine Oculomotor Deficits?
Basic Observation: fixation, saccadic eye movements, difficulty tracking with smooth pursuits, convergence & divergence, decreased ROM, diplopia

ADL Function: hand-eye coordination issues, mobility, reading, measuring, cutting, and pouring

What are interventions for Oculomotor Deficits?
Intervention: Eye movement activities, visuo-motor tasks, scanning tasks, increase endurance during tasks

How would a therapist determine Perception Deficits?
Basic Observation: difficulty scanning, disorganized space, impulsive behavior

ADL Function: loses items, difficulty with grooming & dressing, difficulty navigating in familiar environments

What are interventions for Perception Deficitis?
Intervention: emphasize scanning left and right, integrate spontaneous scanning into ADLs, and occlude one eye at a time

How would a therapist determine Visual Spatial Perception Deficits?
Basic Observation: inability to distinguish space around one's body, objects in relation to body & environment

ADL Function: dressing & self-care, locating objects in environment

What is intervention for Visual Spatial Perception Deficits?
Intervention: have client pick out objects of similar color to the background, modify the environment organizing & labeling, practice scanning & organization to compensate.

What is Agnosia?
impairment in the ability to recognize & identify objects using only visual means, caused by lesion to right occipital lobe

What is Color Agnosia?
inability to recognize or remember specific colors

What is Color Anomia?
inability to name specific colors

What is Object Agnosia?
inability to recognize objects using only vision

What is Prosopagnosia?
inability to recognize or identify a known face or individual

What is Simultanagnosia?
inability to recognize & interpret an entire visual array at a time

What is Stereognosis?
ability to identify everyday objects using tactile properties, no vision

What is Graphesthesia?
ability to identify forms, numbers, letters

What is Autotopagnosia?
inability to identify body parts on self or someone else

What is Finger Agnosia?
inability to recognize which finger was being touched or being used, may display clumsiness with fingers

What is Anosognosia?
lack of recognition or awareness of one's deficits

Allen Cognitive Levels

Discuss Components of Each of Allen's Cognitive Levels

Level 1
Reflexive
Difficulty focusing on external stimuli
May or may not be able to eat or drink
Individual is conscious
Requires 24 hour care
Can attend for a few seconds
Response to external environment is minimal

Level 2
Demonstrates movement
Have postural actions
Can attend 5-10 minutes
Have proprioceptive cues
Individual may assist caregiver with simple tasks
Unable to imitate running stitch (related to assessment)

Level 3
Determine manual actions
Understands tactile cues
Can attend for up to 30-40 minutes
Have repetitive actions
Can repeat actions of others
Demonstrates an understanding of cause and effect
Able to imitate all 3 running stitches (related to assessment)
Cannot follow written directions
Able to help with self-care

Level 4
Goal directed
Independent with self-care
Can live alone
Attends for 45 minutes
Relies heavily on visual cues
Can follow written directions

Can imitate the whip stitch (related to assessment)

Level 5
Exploratory
Understands related cues
Can carry over for several days
Overt (physical) trial and error
Demonstrates Problem solving
Can complete simple craft without written instructions
Anticipates safety
Able to drive
Social bonding occurs
Can imitate single cordovan stitch (related to assessment

Level 6
Plans actions
Understands symbolic cues
Unlimited actions
Premeditated activities
Individual can think of hypothetical situations
Complete mental trial and error problem solving
Can imitate cordovan stitches (related to assessment)

OT Terms

Amelia
An extremely rare birth defect marked by the absence of one or more limbs.

Phocomelia
A developmental anomaly characterized by absence of the upper part of one or more of the limbs so that the feet or hands or both are attached to the trunk.
Caused by thalidomide during pregnancy

Kinesthesia
The sense that detects bodily movement, or weight, of the muscles, tendons, and joints

Dysmetria
The inability or impaired ability to accurately control the range of movement in muscular acts (undershoot/overshoot)

Dysarthria
A condition that results in distorted speech

Akinesia
Inability to initiate movement

Dystonia
Involuntary sustained distorted movement

Chorea
Short duration of rapid, irregular, involuntary movement of face & extremities

Agnosia
Difficulty with recognition of objects through visual input alone
A symptom is Loss of knowledge of objects through sight alone.

Ideational apraxia
The Breakdown in the knowledge of what is to be done or how to perform specific activities.

Ideational apraxia
Physical prompts required
May be step by step or generalized, but are more effective than verbal prompts

Ideomotor apraxia
Loss of access to kinesthetic (bodies movements) memory so that purposeful movements cannot be achieved
Ineffective motor planning

Ideomotor apraxia
Utilizes general verbal and visual cues

Topographical disorientation
Difficulty finding ones way in their surrounding secondary to memory dysfunction or inability to interpret sensory stimuli

Prospective review
Evaluation and approval of proposed intervention plans by 3rd party payers

Utilization review
Review of the resources used within a facility to determine medical necessity and cost efficiency.

Dyspraxia
Difficulty with motor planning in regards to movement and coordination.
Seen with CP, MS, MD, and Parkinson's

Co-contraction
Ability of opposing muscle groups to contract at the same time providing stability around a joint
Push and pull in an arc type motion.

Orthostatic hypotension
Form of hypotension in which a person's blood pressure suddenly falls when the person stands suddenly or stretches (after standing)

Orthostatic hypotension
Symptoms include weakness, light-headedness, cognitive impairment, blurred vision, vertigo, and tremulousness.

Vertigo
Sensation of motion or spinning that is often described as dizziness.
A feeling the world is spinning

Autonomic dysreflexia
Commonly seen in S.I patients

Task oriented group
Goal is to increase member's awareness of feelings, thoughts, needs, and values through the process of choosing, planning, and implementing a group activity.

Topical group
Goal is to improve activity performance through problem solving.
Verbal-based group focuses on the discussion of activities members are currently engaged in or will be engaged in soon.

Instrumental group
Goal is to function at highest level for as long as possible
Individuals with chronic disabilities with no anticipation for improvement

Thematic group
Goal is to assist members in acquiring the knowledge and/or attitudes for a specific set of skills independently

Criterion measure
In conjunction with other data determines rates (such as %) of success

Autonomic dysreflexia
Occurs most often in spinal injury patients above the T6 level. It is a reaction of the ANS to cause an extreme rise in blood pressure caused by noxious stimulus, which must be removed immediately.
Symptoms include throbbing/pounding headache, profuse sweating, and nasal stuffiness and flushed face
A blocked catheter and overfilled urine bag are common precipitants to this complication.

Upper motor neuron lesion injury
Results in general weakness, loss of voluntary muscle control, spasticity and hyperreflexia.

Anoxia
Total decrease in the level of oxygen supply to the organ and the tissues, an extreme form of hypoxia

Splinting and Diagnoses

What splint is used for a Brachial plexus injury?
flail arm splint

What splint is used for Radial nerve palsy?
dynamic wrist splint, finger & thumb extension splint

What splint is used for Median nerve palsy?
C-bar (thenar web spacer) or thumb post splint => Basic
opponens splint, stabilization of first MCP joint

What splint is used for an Ulnar nerve injury?
static/dynamic splint to position MCPs in flexion

What splint is used for a Combined median/ulnar injury?
figure eight or dynamic MCP flexion splint

What splint is used for a Spinal cord C6-C7?
Tenodesis splint

What splint is used for a DeQuervains disease?
Thumb spica splint (includes wrist) IP joint is free, wrist is
commonly in 15* of extension

What splint is used for a Swan Neck?
Silver rings or buttonhole splint

What splint is used for a Boutonniere?
Silver rings or dynamic PIP extension splint

What splint is used for a Carpal tunnel syndrome?
Position wrist cock up
Volor splint in neutral with MAX of 3* ulnar deviation and avoid wrist flexion activities.

What splint is used for a Pronator Teres syndrome?
Elbow splint @ 90* with forearm in neutral

What splint is used for a Cubital tunnel syndrome?
Elbow splint to prevent positions of extreme flexion (especially at night)

What splint is used for a Medial nerve laceration?
Dorsal protection splint with wrist positioned in:
30* of flexion if low lesion
Include elbow (90* flexion) if high lesion
C bar to prevent thumb adduction contractures

What splint is used for an Ulnar nerve laceration?
Dorsal protection splint with wrist positioned in:
30* of flexion if low lesion
Include elbow (90* flexion) if high lesion
MCP flexion block splint

What splint is used for a Radial nerve laceration?
Dynamic extension splint

What is the Kleinert protocol?
Active extension of digits with passive flexion by using rubber band traction.
Uses a dorsal block splint

What is the Duran protocol?
Passive flexion and extension of digits.
Uses a dorsal block splint.

Describe the purpose of the Long opponens splint
Used for preventing radial and ulnar deviation deformities

Describe the purpose of the Swan neck splint
F.O that prevents hyperextension of the PIP joint but allow for full IP flexion

Describe the purpose of the Boutonniere splint
F.O. that immobilizes the PIP in extension (prevents flexion)

Describe the purpose of the Balanced forearm orthosis
Useful with muscle weakness such as Guillan-Barre syndrome, muscular dystrophy and brachial plexus injury.
A MMT above 2 is required & coordination of elbow flexion (can be used with C5 quad)

Describe the purpose of the Overhead suspension sling
Best suited for individual presenting with proximal weakness & MMT of 1/5 to 3/5.

Describe the purpose of the Bilateral soft elbow splints
Fix elbow at 20-30 degrees of flexion when using splint

Describe the purpose of the Wrist cock-up splint

Allows full MCP flexion while maintaining the functional position of the wrist and hand. Uses include resting wrist and hand in acute RA, carpal tunnel syndrome, & to reduce spasticity.

Describe the purpose of the Resting hand splint

Static wrist-hand orthosis used to immobilize the wrist, fingers and thumb. Used b/c MCPs and IPs are kept stretched (minimizing future joint contractures)

Describe the purpose of the Static splint

No moving parts, utilized for external support, prevention of motion, aligning joints for healing or reducing pain.

Describe the purpose of the Dynamic splint

Moving parts are included, utilized to increase passive ROM, assist weak motions or substitute for lost motion

Describe the purpose of the Serial splint

Utilized to achieve a slow, progressive increase in ROM by progressive remolding, as well as reduces tone and contractures in burns.

What is the treatment protocol for Dupuytrens disease?

Requires extension splint initially 24 hours a day, 7 days a week. Scar management including scar massage, scar pad and compression garment.

What is the treatment protocol for Lateral/Medial epicondylitis?

Conservative treatment includes elbow strap and wrist splint, ice and deep friction massage, and stretching.

Describe the purpose of the Plaster cylindrical splint
Encourages a STATIC stretch of the PIP joint contracture.

Describe the purpose of the Dynamic outrigger splint
Form of PIP extension

What is the treatment protocol for CRPS?
Volar wrist immobilization splint during functional activities as tolerated
Circumferential wrist splint to help avoid pressure/edema.

What is the treatment protocol for DeQuervains disease?
Long forearm based or radial gutter splint with wrist in 15* of extension.

Pediatric Milestones

FINE MOTOR & SELF CARE
1 year to 15 months
Finger to palm translation (picking up a coin)

1 1/2 year to 21 months
Recognizes shapes, thinks before doing
Operates a mechanical toy

21 months to 2 years

Can match shapes (circle, square, etc.)
Manipulate objects (i.e. shape sorter)

2 to 2.5 years
Builds a block tower
Palm to finger translation and simple rotation

2 years
Pulls down pants
Finds armholes in pullover

2.5 years
Unbuttons large buttons

3 to 3.5 years
Shift (separating paper)
Pullover shirt with min A
Independently pulls down pants
Buttons large buttons
Unzips/zips with setup

3.5 to 4 years
Finds front of clothing & dresses with supervision
Builds a block tower of 9 cubes
Organizes by size and constructs mental images

4 years
Pulls off pullover independently
Zips jacket
Buckles belt or shoe
Shoes/socks min A.

4.5 years
Able to put belt in loops

5 years
Dresses unsupervised; ties knots

6 years
Ties bows

6 to 7 years
In hand manipulation & complex rotation

EATING
6.5 to 7 months
Self- feeding with a cracker

7 to 8 months
Mastication of soft and mashed foods with diagonal jaw movement

9 months
Holding and banging a spoon
Able to drink from cup
Jaw not firm

9.5 months
Stirring with a spoon
Finger feeds portion of meal

12 to 14 months

Bringing a filled spoon to mouth but spills food by inverting spoon before it reaches mouth

15 to 18 months
Scoops food with spoon and brings to mouth

1 year
Jaw is firm
Rotary chewing
Good bite on hard cookie

2 years
Able to chew most meats and raw veggies

Pediatrics UE development

Reaching: Newborn
Reaching skills
Visual regard with swiping/batting

Reaching: 4 months
Hands come together at midline with bilateral reaching
Shoulders abducted with partial internal rotation
Forearm pronation and full finger extension

Reaching: 6 months
Increased dissociation
Less shoulder abduction and internal rotation
Hand is more open

Reaching: 9 months
Trunk stability improves

Shoulder flexion slight external rotation
Forearm supination
Slight wrist extension

Grasping: natal
No voluntary grasp or visual attention

Grasping: 3 months
No attempt to grasp
Visually attends to object

Grasping: 6 months
Raking and contacting object

Grasping: 7 months
Inferior scissors grasp: raking into palm with adducted totally
flexed thumb and all flexed fingers

Grasping: 8 months
Scissors grasp: between thumb and side of curled index finger,
distal thumb joint slightly flexed, proximal thumb joint extended

Grasping: 9 months
Inferior pincer grasp: between ventral side thumb and index
finger, distal thumb joint extended, beginning of thumb
opposition

Grasping: 10 months
Pincer grasp: between distal pads of thumb and index finger,
distal thumb joint slightly flexed. Thumb in opposition

Grasping: 12 months
Fine pincer grasp: between fingertips or fingernails, distal thumb joint flexed

Grasp cube: neonate
Visually attends to object, grasp reflexive

Grasp cube: 3 months
Visually attends and may swipe.
Sustained grasp possible but only upon contact, no thumb involvement, wrist flexed

Grasp cube: 4 months
Primitive squeeze grasp: visually attends, may approach if within 1 in, contact in hand pulling object back to squeeze against other hand or body, no thumb involvement

Grasp cube: 5 months
Palmar grasp: fingers on top surface, object presses into center of palm with thumb adducted

Grasp cube: 6 months
radial palmar grasp: fingers on far side of object press it against opposed thumb and radial side of palm with wrist flexed. Wrist straight (7 months)

Grasp cube: 8 months
Radial digital grasp: object held with opposed thumb and fingertips. Space visible between. Wrist extended (9 months)

Releasing: 1-4 months
Involuntary release

Releasing: 5-6 months
Two hand transfer

Releasing: 6-7 months
One hand transfer

Releasing: 7-9 months
Voluntary release

Manipulating: 12-15 months
Finger to palm translation

Manipulating: 2-2 1/2 yrs
Palm to finger translation

Manipulating: 3-3 1/2 yrs
Shift: linear movement object on the finger surface (separating two pieces of paper)

Manipulating: 2-2 1/2 years
Simple rotation: turning or rolling object 90 degrees or less

Manipulating: 6-7 years
Complex rotation: rotation of object 360 degrees (turning a pencil to erase)

Manipulating: 6-7 years
In hand manipulation with stabilization: several objects held in the hand and manipulation of object occurs while simultaneously stabilizing others

Pre writing: 1- 1 1/2 years
Palmar-supinate grasp: held with fisted hand, wrist slightly flexed and slightly supinated. arm moves as unit

Pre-writing: 2-3 years
Digital pronate grasp: held with fingers, wrist neutral with slight ulnar deviation and forearm pronation. Arm moves as unit

Pre-writing: 3 1/2-4 years
Static tripod grasp: grasped proximally with continuous adjustments by other hand, no fine localized movements. Hand moves as a unit

Pre-writing: 4 1/2-6 years
Dynamic tripod grasp: held with precise opposition. MCP joints stabilized during fine, localized movements of PIP joints

Scissors: 2-3 years
Shows an interest in scissors. Holds and snips with scissors. Opens and closes scissors in controlled fashion

Scissors: 3-4 years
Manipulates scissors in a forward motion
Coordinates the lateral direction of scissors
Cuts a straight forward line
Cuts simple geometric shapes

Scissors: 3 1/2-4 1/2 years
Cuts circles

Scissors: 4-6 years
Cuts simple figure shapes

Scissors: 6-7 years
Cuts complex figure shapes

MET Levels

Class I
Max METs 6.5
No limits to activity
No complaints

Class II
Max METs 4.5
Slight activity limit
Comfort at rest
Ordinary activity results in fatigue, pain, and dyspnea

Class III
Max METs 3.0
Marked limitation - comfort at rest, less than ordinary activity
result in fatigue, palpitations, dyspnea and angina pain

Class IV
Max METs 1.5
Inability to carry out physical activity without discomfort
Increased discomfort with activity

Stage I
1.0-1.4 METs sitting: self feeding, hand and face wash, transfers; progressively increase sitting tolerance; supine: exercise to all extremities; sitting: exercise only to neck and lower extremities; Include deep breathing exercises; reading, table games and light handwork

Stage II
1.4-2.0 METs Unlimited sitting: self-bathing, shaving, grooming and dressing; ambulation at slow pace in room as tolerated; exercise to all extremities while sitting; progressively increase number of repetitions; NO ISOMETRICS; leisure crafts while sitting; crafts, painting, knitting, sewing, mosaics and embroidery

Stage III
2.0-3.0 METs; sitting showering in warm water; homemaking tasks with brief standing periods to transfer light items, ironing; wheelchair mobility, limited distances; standing and exercise to all extremities and trunk, progressively increasing the number reps; may include (1) balance exercises; (2) light mat activities without resistance; begin progressive ambulation at 0% grade; leisure activities include card playing, crafts, piano, machine sewing and typing

Stage IV
3.0-3.5 METs; standing total washing, dressing, shaving, grooming, showering in warm water; kitchen & homemaking

activities while practicing energy conservation techniques (light vacuuming, dusting and sweeping, washing light clothes); unlimited distance walking 0% grade; standing continue all previous exercise progressively increasing number of reps and speed of reps; leisure activities include candlepin bowling, canoeing (slow), golf putting, light gardening and driving

Stage V
3.5-4.0 METs; standing; washing dishes, washing clothes, ironing, hanging light clothes, and making beds; exercise (same as previous); ambulation 2.5 mph on level surface, stairs to patient tolerance, cycling up to 8 mph without resistance, leisure swimming (slowly), light carpentry, golfing (using cart), light home repairs

Stage VI
4.0 -5.0 METs; standing; showering in HOT water; hanging or wringing clothes, mopping, stripping and making beds, raking; ambulation 3.5 mph on level surfaces; stairs as tolerated by patient; treadmill 1.5 mph at 5-6% grade; 3.5 mph at 0% grade; cycling 10 mph without resistance; 10-15 lbs. weights in multi-rep upper and lower body reps

EXAMPLES OF ACTIVITIES & RELATED METs
1.5-2 METs
desk work, driving, typing, electric calculating machine operation; standing, walking 1 mph, motorcycling, playing cards and sewing, knitting

2-3 METs
auto-repair, radio & TV repair, janitorial work, typing, bartending, level walking 2 mph, bicycling 5 mph, riding lawn mower, billiards, bowling skeet, shuffleboard, wood working, power boat driving, golf, canoeing 2.5 mph, horseback riding (walk pace), playing piano and other musical instruments

3-4 METs

brick layering, plastering, wheelbarrow (230 lb. load), machine assembly, trailer truck in traffic, welding, cleaning windows, walking 3 mph, cycling 6 mph, horse shoe pitching, volleyball, golf, archery, sailing, fly fishing, horseback riding (up to trot), badminton, pushing light power mower, energetic musician

4-5 METs

painting, masonry, paperhanging, light carpentry, walking 3.5 mph, cycling 8 mph, table tennis, golf, dancing, badminton, tennis, raking leaves, hoeing, calisthenics

5-6 METs

digging garden, shoveling light earth, walking 4 mph, cycling 10 mph, canoeing 4 mph, horseback (posting to trot), stream fishing, ice or roller-skating 9 mph

6-7 METs

shoveling 10 min (22lbs), walking 5 mph, cycling 11 mph, badminton, tennis, splitting wood, snow shoveling, manual lawn mowing, square dancing, light downhill skiing, ski touring (2.5 mph), water skiing

7-8 METs

digging ditches, carrying 175 lbs., sawing hardwood, jogging 5 mph, cycling 12 mph, horseback riding (gallop), vigorous downhill skiing, basketball, mountain climbing, ice hockey, canoeing (5 mph), touch football, paddleball

8-9 METs

shoveling 10 min (31 lbs.), running 5.5 mph, cycling 13 mph, ski touring 4 mph, squash, handball, fencing, basketball

10+ METs
shoveling 10 min (35 lbs.), running 6 mph, skiing 5+ mph,
handball, squash

Wheelchair Measurements

What are adult standard Wheelchair dimensions?
width 18
depth 16
height 20

What are narrow adult Wheelchair dimensions?
width 16
depth 16
height 20

What are junior Wheelchair dimensions?
width 16
depth 16
height 18.5

How is Wheelchair seat depth determined?
Measure both LE
Take greatest length
Subtract 2 inches
Measure from posterior portion of the buttocks to the popliteal
fossa then subtract 2 inches

How is Wheelchair seat width determined?
Measure the widest point across the hips and thighs to allow for maximal space
Add 2 inches

How is Wheelchair seat height determined?
With knees and ankles positioned at 90 degrees; measure from distal thigh to heel with a 2" clearance from the floor

What are wrap around arm rests?
Space savers
Reduces overall width by 1"

24-26" is the average Wheelchair what?
Average Wheelchair width

32" is the average what?
Minimum doorway clearance

36" is the ideal what?
Ideal doorway clearance

What does removing doorstops do to the doorway?
adds 3/4"

What do offset hinges do to the doorway?
Adds 1 1/2-2"

What is the turning space for a Wheelchair?
5' x 5' (60" x 60") – 360 degrees

What is the maximum height an individual can reach from his/her chair?
48"

What is the maximum reachable height for countertops?
31"

What is the minimum space requirement for parking?
4' aisle

What is the minimum width of pathways and walkways?
48"

What is the ramp slope requirement?
1" vertical rise to 12"

What are the required railing measurements?
29-36"

How high are curbs on ramps?
4" high

How long is required for a landing for turning a Wheelchair?
48'

How long is required for a 90-degree turn?
4' x 4'

How long is required for a 180-degree turn?
4' x 8'

What does leaning forward indicate?
Armrests are too low

What does shoulder elevation indicate?
Armrests are too high

What are adult Wheelchair dimensions?
18" W x 16" D x 20" H

What are narrow adult Wheelchair dimensions?
16" W x 16" D x 20" H

What are slim adult Wheelchair dimensions?
14" W x 16" D x 20" H

What is the measurement of a hemi/low-seat?
17.5" H

What are junior Wheelchair dimensions?
16" W x 16" D x 18.5" H

What are child Wheelchair dimensions?
14" W x 11.5" D x 18.75" H

What are tiny tot Wheelchair dimensions?
12" W x 11/5" D x 19.5" H

Rancho Levels

Level 1
No response total assist needed
Unresponsive to all stimuli

Level 2
Generalized response total assist
Non-purposeful
Non-specific reactions to stimuli
Responds to pain (may be delayed)

Level 3
Localized response total assist
Responds to some commands
May respond to discomfort

Level 4
Confused, agitated
Needs max assist
Disoriented
Inappropriate behavior frequent
Short attention span

Level 5
Confused, inappropriate, non-agitated
Needs max assist
Appears alert

Responds to simple commands

Level 6
Confused appropriate moderate assist
Able to attend to highly familiar tasks in non-distracting
environment for 30 minutes

Level 7
Automatic and appropriate response minimal assistance for
daily living skills
Insight, judgment and problem solving poor

Level 8
Purposeful, appropriate
Standby assist
Poor tolerance for stress
Depression
Some abstract reasoning difficulties

Level 9
Purposeful, appropriate
Standby assist on request
Shifts back and forth between tasks and completes in at least 2
consecutive hours

Level 10
Purposeful, appropriate
Independent
Able to handle multiple tasks in all environments

MMT and Range of Motion

RANGE OF MOTION FOR UE
Shoulder
Flexion: 0-170 degrees
Extension: 0-60
Abduction: 0-170
Adduction: 0
Horizontal Abduction: 0-40
Horizontal Adduction: 0-130
Internal Rotation: 0-60/70
External Rotation: 0-80/90

Elbow
Flexion: 0-135/150
Extension: 0

Forearm
Pronation: 0-80/90
Supination: 0-80/90

Wrist
Flexion: 0-80
Extension: 0-70
Ulnar Deviation: 0-30
Radial Deviation: 0-20

Thumb
DIP Flexion: 0-80/90
MP Flexion: 0-50
Adduction: 0
Palmer Abduction: 0-50
Radial Abduction: 0-50

Opposition: composite motion

Fingers
MP Flexion: 0-90
MP Hyperextension: 0-15/45
PIP Flexion: 0-110
DIP Flexion: 0-80
Abduction: 0-25

MMT
Grade 0
No muscle contraction is seen or felt

Grade 1 (Trace)
Contraction can be felt, but there is no motion

Grade 2- (Poor minus)
Part moves through incomplete ROM with gravity decreased

Grade 2 (Poor)
Part moves through complete ROM with gravity decreased

Grade 2+ (Poor Plus)
Part moves through incomplete ROM (less than 50%) against gravity or through complete ROM with gravity decreased with slight resistance

Grade 3- (Fair minus)
Part moves through incomplete ROM (more than 50%) against gravity

Grade 3 (Fair)
Part moves through complete ROM against gravity

Grade 3+ (Fair Plus)
Part moves through complete ROM against gravity and slight resistance

Grade 4 (Good)
Part moves through complete ROM against gravity and moderate resistance

Grade 5 (Normal)
Part moves through complete ROM against gravity and full resistance

Spinal Cord Levels & Injury Concepts

C2
Adam's Apple to back of head

C3
Clavicle

C4
Tops of shoulders

C5
Biceps

C6

Radial forearm to thumb & pointer finger

C7
3 finger

C8
4 & 5 finger

T1
Ulnar forearm

T2
Armpits

T3
Body of the sternum

T4
Nipple line

T5
Where bra wire would lie

T6-T9
Ribs

T10
Belly button

T11
Top of underwear line

T12
Hipbones

L1
Groin to interior thighs

L2
Interior thighs

L3
Knees

L4
Tibia

L5
Fibula to first 3 toes

S1
Last 2 toes to middle of calf

S2
Back of knees and thighs

S3
Circle around butt

S4-5
Anal canal

What is Central Cord Syndrome?
(center of cord) resulting from hyperextension injuries
Presenting as more UE deficits vs. LE deficits

What is Brown-Sequard Syndrome (Lateral Damage)?
(one side of the cord) resulting in ipsilateral spastic paralysis
Loss of position sense, contralateral loss of pain, thermal sense

What is Anterior Cord Syndrome?
Caused by flexion injuries
Loss bilaterally of motor function

Loss of pain, temp & touch sensation.
Prop is preserved.

What is Conus Medullaris Syndrome?

Injury of the sacral cord & lumbar nerve roots resulting in LE motor & sensory loss & arelfexic bowel & bladder (atonic or flaccid)

What is Cauda Equina Syndrome?

Flaccid paralysis with no spinal reflex activity

What is Tetraplegia (quadriplegia)?

C1 to T1.
Any degree of paralysis of the four limbs and trunk musculature.

What is Paraplegia?

T2 to S5.
Loss of sensory & motor control of the chest, stomach, hips, legs and feet. (paralysis of the LE's)

Discuss Injury to Each Below Level

C1-C3

Limited movement of head and neck

Breathing: Depends on a ventilator for breathing.

Communication: Talking is sometimes difficult, very limited or impossible. Communication can be accomplished independently with a mouth stick and assistive technologies like a computer for speech or typing.

Effective verbal communication allows the individual with SCI to direct caregivers in the person's daily activities, like bathing, dressing, personal hygiene, transferring as well as bladder and bowel management.

Daily tasks: Assistive technology allows for independence in tasks such as turning pages, using a telephone and operating lights and appliances.

Mobility: Can operate an electric wheelchair by using a head control, mouth stick, or chin control. A power tilt wheelchair also for independent pressure relief.

C3-C4

Usually has head and neck control.

Individuals at C4 level may shrug their shoulders.

Breathing: May initially require a ventilator for breathing, usually adjust to breathing full-time without ventilator assistance.

Communication: Normal.

Daily tasks: With specialized equipment, some may have limited independence in feeding and independently operate an adjustable bed with an adapted controller.

C5

Typically has head and neck control, can shrug shoulder and has shoulder control. Can bend his/her elbows and turn palm. Has bicep use.

Daily tasks: Independence with eating, drinking, face washing, brushing of teeth, face shaving and hair care after assistance in setting up specialized equipment.

Health care: Can manage their own health care by doing self-assist coughs and pressure reliefs by leaning forward or side -to-side.

Mobility: May have strength to push a manual wheelchair for short distances over smooth surfaces. A power wheelchair with hand controls is typically used for daily activities.

Driving may be possible after being evaluated by a qualified professional to determine special equipment needs

C6

Has movement in head, neck, shoulders, arms and wrists. Can shrug shoulders, bend elbows, turn palms up and down and extend wrists. Has tendonesis grasp.

Daily tasks: With help of some specialized equipment, can perform with greater ease and independence, daily tasks of feeding, bathing, grooming, personal hygiene and dressing. May independently perform light housekeeping duties.

Health care: Can independently do pressure reliefs, skin checks and turn in bed.

Mobility: Some individuals can independently do transfers but often require a sliding board. Can use a manual wheelchair for daily activities but may use power wheelchair for greater ease of independence.

C7

Has similar movement as an individual with C6, with added ability to straighten his/her elbows. Has triceps function

Daily tasks: Able to perform household duties. Need fewer adaptive aids in independent living.

Health care: Able to do wheelchair pushups for pressure reliefs.

Mobility: Daily use of manual wheelchair. Can transfer with greater ease.

C8-T1

Has added strength and precision of fingers that result in limited or natural hand function.

Daily tasks: Can live independently without assistive devices in feeding, bathing, grooming, oral and facial hygiene, dressing, bladder management and bowel management.

Mobility: Uses manual wheelchair. Can transfer independently.

T2-T6

Has normal motor function in head, neck, shoulders, arms, hands and fingers. Has increased use of rib and chest muscles, or trunk control.

Daily tasks: Should be totally independent with all activities.

Mobility: A few individuals are capable of limited walking with extensive bracing. This requires extremely high energy and puts stress on the upper body, offering no functional advantage. Can lead to damage of upper joints.

T7-T12

Has added motor function from increased abdominal control.

Daily tasks: Able to perform unsupported seated activities.

Mobility: Same as T2-T6

Health care: Has improved cough effectiveness.

L1-L5
Has additional return of motor movement in hips and knees.

Mobility: Walking can be a viable function, with the help of specialized leg and ankle braces. Lower levels walk with greater ease with the help of assistive devices.

S1-S5
Depending on level of injury, there are various degrees of return of voluntary bladder, bowel and sexual functions.

Mobility: Increased ability to walk with fewer or no supportive devices.

A
Complete, no sensory or motor function is preserved S4-S5.

B
Incomplete, sensory but no motor function is preserved below level of injury.

C
Incomplete, sensory & motor function is preserved below level of injury, muscle grade less than 3/5.

D
Incomplete, sensory & motor function is preserved below level of injury, muscle grade greater than 3/5.

E
Normal, sensory & motor function is normal.

What are specific precautions & contraindications with SCI?
Decreased vital capacity
Autonomic dysreflexia
Orthostatic hypotension
Pressure ulcers
Bowel & bladder dysfunction
Thermal dysregulation
Pain
Fatigue
Deep vein thrombosis
Spasticity & spasm
Heterotopic ossification
Osteoporosis
Decreased motor skill for sexual intimacy

What is Autonomic Dysreflexia?
A potentially life-threatening situation for SCI patients, which requires immediate attention
Episodic high blood pressure leading to: throbbing headaches, profuse sweating, and nasal stuffiness, flushing of the skin above the level of the lesion, bradycardia, apprehension and anxiety

Causes: painful stimuli, tight clothing, hanging limbs cutting off blood circulation, blocked urinary catheter, stool impaction

SCI Therapeutic Intervention

C1-C3

What movements can a C1-C3 utilize?
chew, swallow, talk, and blow

What is C1-C3 techniques/ equipment for self care?
ventilator

What are long term goals for self care C1-C3?
Directs other for all applicable care including pressure relief, skin, precautions, upper extremity ROM techniques, equipment maintenance, activity and equipment s/u procedures, upper extremity positioning in bed and Wheelchair

What are C1, C3 techniques/ equipment for mobility?
Wheelchair (electronically controlled electric Wheelchair can use sip and puff or head control, appropriate seating system for positioning and safety)

Pressure relief (electronically controlled recline or tilt mechanism

What are C1, C3 communication techniques/ equipment?
Word processing- computer using infrared head pointer, single or dual action switches, or mouth stick
Telephone-speaker phone, adapted for automatic dialing

What is a C1, C3 long-term goal for communication?
Minimal assistance

What are C1, C3 recreation equipment/ techniques?
Games- computer/ electronic
Art- mouth stick painting with s/u
Reading-electronic page-turner or turn pages with mouth stick

Vocation- computer with head point, switches, or mouth stick

What are C1, C3 long-term goals for recreation?
Minimum assistance with all devices/ techniques

C4
What movements can a C4 do?
Respiration
Scapular elevation

What are C4 techniques or equipment for self care?
Feeding- long straw with straw holder

What are C4 techniques or equipment for mobility?
Wheelchair - electronically controlled wheelchair using sip and puff, cin switch, or head control
Pressure relief- electronically controlled wheelchair with power recline/tilt mechanism

What is a C4 Long term goals for mobility?
Independent with wheelchair propulsion inside on hard level surfaces, independent with supervision outdoors on hard surfaces, dependent/directs others for assist with architectural barriers, independent with power recline/tilt wheelchair

What is a C4 long-term goal for self care?
Minimal assistance for drinking
Directs others for all applicable care

C4 fully innervated level and key muscles are what?
diaphragm and trapezius

C5

C5 last fully innervated level and key muscles are which ones?
biceps, brachialis, brachioradialis, supinator, Infraspinatus, deltoid

What movements can a C5 do?
Elbow flexion and supination
Shoulder external rotation
Shoulder abduction to 80-90
Gravity provides shoulder adduction, pronation, and internal rotation

What are C5 self care techniques/ equipment for feeding?
Mobile arm support or suspension sling
Dorsal wrist splint with ucuff
Dycem to stabilize plate, plate guard or scoop dish
Stabilized cup or cup holder
Long straw with straw holder
Angled spoon or fork,

What are C5 long-term goals?
A ratchet splint can be used to increase level of functional independence

What are C5 long-term goals for self care?
Minimal assistance for these tasks

What are C5 Long term goals for dressing?
Mod A with UE
Max A with LE

What are C5 grooming/bathing techniques/equipment?
Wash mitts
Quad grip hairbrush
Makeup for ucuff
LH sponge

What are C5 mobility techniques and equipment?
Wheelchair -hand controlled power wheelchair, manual
wheelchair with projection knobs
Pressure relief- "power recline" or tilt wheelchair with use of
elbow or head switches

What are C5 Long term goals for mobility?
Independent with propulsion inside on hard level surfaces
I/S outdoors on hard surfaces
directs others for assist with architectural barriers

What are C5 communication techniques and equipment?
Word processing- typing stick placed in dorsal wrist splint with
ucuff
Writing- long writing orthosis
Phone-push button speaker, typing stick to press buttons
Reading- turn pages manually using book holder and typing stick
in dorsal wrist splint with ucuff

What are C5 Communication Long term goals?
Min A with these tasks required

C6
C6 last fully innervated level and key muscles are what?

pectoralis major, serratus anterior, lattisimus dorsal, pronator
Teres, radial wrist extensors

What movements can C6 movements do?
Shoulder flexion
Reach outward
Shoulder internal rotation and extension
Shoulder adduction
More respiratory reserve
Pronation
Wrist extension (Tenodesis grasp)

What are C6 Feeding techniques or equipment?
Ucuff
Rocker knife or sharp paring knife,
Does not need long handled straw
May use cup with long handle
Does not need plate guard (mod I)

What are C6 grooming techniques or equipment?
Tenodesis grasp with adaptive equipment (mod I)

What are C6 bathing techniques or equipment?
Bench
Must reach facet (min A)

What are C6 bowel and bladder care techniques or equipment?_
Insert suppositories with ae
Adaptive handles
Independent with toilet transfer, applying condom
Self catherization - adaptive clamp for drainage bag (male- min A, female- max A)

What are C6 dressing techniques or equipment?
Dressing in bed
Uses button hook
Uses zipper pull
Clothes should be correct size or larger (UE- mod I, LE- min-max A)

What are C6 wheelchair mobility techniques or equipment?
Pushes manual wheelchair with friction material or rims or projection knobs
An electric wheelchair may be required for long distances (Independent in propelling on level surfaces, min A on uneven surfaces)

What are C6 transfer techniques and equipment?
Uses a transfer board and partial depression or swivel transfer (independent)

What are C6 bed transfer techniques and equipment?
Possible loops at bottom of bed

What are C6 long-term goals for bed transfers?
Mod I for rolling supine to long sitting
Mod A for proning, paddling, and positioning

What are C6 vehicle techniques and equipment?
Drive using hand controls with adapted steering wheel (mod I)

What are C6 pressure relief goals?
Independent side to side

What are C6 communication techniques?
Word processing- ucuff for Tenodesis grasp to hold typing stick
Writing-uses Tenodesis grasp to hold pen or short writing orthosis
Telephone- uses any phone or phone holder or uses Tenodesis grasp to hold receiver
(mod I with all tasks)

What are C6 recreation techniques and equipment?
Can turn on and off radio/ TV
Can play table games with adaptations
Can participate in some Wheelchair sports

What are C6 vocation techniques and equipment?
Cannot use hand tools that require strength
Electronic office machines are well suited to these patients
Homemaking can do light cooking and cleaning, needs a Wheelchair accessible kitchen (light work min A, heavy work- max A)

C7
C7 fully innervated level and key muscles are what?
triceps, extrinsic finger extensors, flexor carpi radialis

What movements can a C7 do?
Elbow extension
Active finger extension (Tenodesis grasp)
Wrist flexion

What are C7 dressing, bathing, bowel/ bladder techniques and equipment?
Buttonhook only
Wheelchair dressing

Same as C6 only is easier

What is C7 mobility techniques/ equipment?
Manual wheelchair
Uses modified car

What are C7 long-term goals for mobility?
Independent with propulsion over flat surfaces and inclines
Independent for rough terrain
Doors: mod I,
Independent with pushups for pressure relief
Min A with padding and positioning
Independent for transfers
Mod I for modified car transfers

C8
C8, T1 key muscles are which?
Intrinsic, including thumb, ulnar wrist flexors and extensors,
extrinsic finger and thumb flexors, extrinsic thumb extensor

What are C8, T1 movements?
Full UE control, including FMC and grasp

**What are C8, T1 self care, mobility, and communication
techniques and equipment?**
Same as C7, but easier
Mod I

T6
T6 key muscles are which?
Top half of intercostal, long muscles of the back

What are movements can T6 do?

Increased endurance due to larger respiratory reserve
Pectoral girdle stabilized for heavy lifting

What are T6 mobility techniques and equipment?
Uses full braces and standing aid for physiological standing only
Can ambulate with great difficulty on level surfaces
(independent)

What are T6 vocation techniques and equipment?
Can work with tools and do fairly heavy lifting and sedentary
position

T12
T12 key muscles are which?
full innervation of intercostal, abdominal muscle

What movements can a T12 do?
Better endurance
Better trunk control

What are T12 self care and mobility techniques or equipment?
For work, sports, and housekeeping:
      Mobility- uses Wheelchair for energy conservation
      Ambulates with difficulty using long leg braces and
crutches
      Can use ride on snow plow, grass cutter, etc., with hand
controls (Independent)

L4
L4 key muscles_____
low back muscles, hip flexors, quadriceps

What movements can a L4 movement do?
Hip flexion
Knee extension

What are L4 mobility techniques and equipment?
Uses canes to prevent deforming effects of degenerate arthritis
Wheelchair might be convenient at home

What are components to L4 bowel and bladder care?
Control is not voluntary

Rood Facilitation Techniques

What is Slow stroking?
An inhibitory technique used to relax hyper-kinetic (overactive muscles) patients

What is Slow rolling/rocking?
Quite effective in inhibiting general muscle hyper tonicity (rigidity or spasticity) Where as fast rocking is contra-indicative because it increases the spasticity.

Neutral warmth & slow rolling for relaxation, and stimulation for reciprocal movement patterns is useful for what disease?
Parkinson's

First stability pattern an OT should facilitate because it is essential for head control is what?
Neck co-contraction

What is High frequency vibration?
Facilitory technique to increase extensor tone

What is Quick ice?
Facilitory technique in which client should try and do opposite reflexively of what therapist does (stimulates muscle)

What is Tendon tapping?
Facilitory technique that increases muscle tone

What does Noxious stimulation or odors do?
Stimulation that is painful is a facilitory technique that helps normalize flaccid muscles.

What do Perfume or pleasant odors do?
Inhibitory technique that helps normalize hypertonic or spastic muscles

What does Constant pressure do?
(Deep pressure as well) The rigid field of an orthokinetic cuff would be inhibitory

What are Facilitory techniques?
Light rapid brushing
Change in environment such as turning on lights
Tapping
Quick stretch
Heavy joint compression
Noxious odors
Painful stimuli

Aimed to stimulate
"Come alive" or maintain control of a muscle group

What are Inhibitory techniques?
Change in environment such as turning of the lights
Gentle shaking of upper limb
Slow rocking
Deep pressure
Slow stroking
Neutral warmth
Aimed to quiet/relax/dampen overactive muscle groups

What is Heavy joint compression?
A facilitory technique applied manually and longitudinally
through a joint in a weight bearing position.

Wrapping a person or a specific body part in a blanket will result in a relaxation response is called what?
Neutral warmth

What does a Maintained stretch do?
Inhibit spastic muscles when done correctly

To gain trunk stability and flexion responses the therapist should do?
Supine Withdrawal

To elicit lateral trunk responses for those dominated by tonic reflexes the therapist should?
Roll to side lying

To elicit Isometric contraction of extensors and ABDs the therapist should do?
Pivot Prone

What develops head control?
Neck co-contraction

To inhibit tonic neck reflexes and provides trunk and proximal limb stability the therapist should use?
Prone on elbows

What should the therapist do to develop limb and trunk co-contraction patterns for crawling?
Quadruped

What should the therapist do to promote static-active weight shifting that increases strength in hips and co contraction in upper body?
Static standing

PNF (Proprioceptive Neuromuscular Facilitation)

Define D1
Starts on same side of body (L hand starts on left side, R hand starts on R side) and moves to contralateral side

Define D2
Starts on opposite side of body and moves to same side.

What is Rhythmical Rotation?
Mobility
Passive technique to decrease hypertonia
Relaxation will increase ROM

What is Rhythmic Initiation?
Mobility
Assist initiating movement when hypertonia exists
Movements must be slow and rhythmical to reduce hypertonia

What are Repeated Contractions?
Mobility
Initiate movement and sustain a contraction though the ROM
Strengthening

What does Contract-Relax do?
Mobility
Increase ROM

What does Hold-Relax do?
Mobility
Isometric contraction to increase ROM
Used for patients that present with pain

What is Slow Reversal?
Stability
Controlled mobility
Slow & resisted concentric contractions of agonists and
antagonists
Improves control of movement and posture

Glascow Coma Scale

Best Verbal Response (V)
Oriented=5
Confused=4
Inappropriate words=3
Incomprehensible Sound=2
None=1

Best Motor Response (M)
Obey commands=6
Localizes to pain=5
Withdraws from pain=4
Flexion in response to pain=3
Extension in response to pain=2
No motor response= 1

Best Eye Response (E)
Eye opening spontaneously=4
Eye opening to speech=3
Eye opening in response to pain= 2
No eye opening=1

Pre-Writing Skills

What is a Palmar-supinated grasp?
Held with fisted hand in a power-like grasp
Extends out from the little finger (ulnar) side of hand arm moves
as a unit
1 to 1-1/2 years
What is a Digital-pronated grasp?

Essentially same as palmar-supinated, with index finger
extended along the pencil, and forearm pronated, arm moves as
a unit
2-3 years

What is a Static Tripod Posture grasp?
Held with crude approximation of thumb, index, middle fingers,
ring and little fingers only slightly flexed
Grasped proximally with continued adjustments by other hand
No fine localized movements of digital components
Hand moves as unit
3 and 1/2 to 4 years

What is a Dynamic Tripod posture grasp?
Held with precise opposition of distal phalanges of thumb,
index, and middle fingers, ring and little fingers flexed to form a
stable arch
Wrist slightly extended, grasped distally, MCP joints stabilized
during fine localized movements of PIP joints
4 and 1/2 to 6 years old

Erik Erikson Stages of Development

Basic trust vs. mistrust
The infant/baby realizes that survival and comfort needs will be
met
Hope is integrated into the personality
(birth to 18 months)

Autonomy vs. doubt and shame
The child realizes that he/she can control bodily functions

Self-controlled will is integrated into the personality
(2 to 4 years)

Initiative vs. guilt
The child gains social skills and a gender role identity
A sense of purpose is integrated into the personality
(preschool age)

Industry vs. inferiority
The child gains a sense of security through peers and gains
mastery over activity of his/her age group
A feeling of competency is integrated into the personality
(elementary school age)

Self-identity vs. role diffusion
The teenager begins to make choices about adult roles
With the resolution of this identity crisis a sense of fidelity or
membership with society is integrated into the personality
(teenage years)

Intimacy and solidarity vs. isolation
The young adult establishes an intimate relationship with a
partner and family
The capacity to love is achieved
(young adulthood)

Generativity vs. self-absorption
The adult finds security in the contribution of his/her chosen
personal/professional roles
The capacity to care is achieved
(middle adulthood)

Integrity vs. despair
The mature adult reflects on his/her own value
Shares with the younger generation the knowledge gained
Wisdom is acquired
(maturity)

Hip Fractures & Replacements

Precautions:
No hip flexion greater than 90 degrees (posterolateral approach)
No internal rotation (posterolateral approach)
No adduction/crossing legs (anterolateral/posterolateral approach)
No external rotation (anterolateral approach)
No external (anterolateral approach)

What is a HEMOVAC?
It is for drainage and is in place 2 days after surgery

What are balanced suspensions used for?
To support the affected leg in the first post operative days
May be removed for exercise

When might a reclining wheel chair be used?
A Wheelchair with an adjustable backrest that allows for reclining is used for patients who have a hip flexion precaution when sitting

What is a sequential compression device (SCD)?
Used post operatively to reduce the risk of DVT

Inflatable, external leggings that provide intermittent pneumatic compression to the legs

What is a knee immobilizer?
It provides support to the knee when moving in and out of bed and ambulating

What is the prosterolateral approach to:
Sitting on a chair?
Do not lean forward when sitting down
Standing from a chair?
Extend the operative leg and push off the armrest

What kind of chairs should be avoided?
Low chairs
Soft chairs
Reclining chairs
Rocking chairs

Assessments

Which assessments are used for ADLs?
Kohlman Evaluation of Living Skills
Bay Area Functional Performance Evaluation
Independent Living Scales Evaluation
Independent Living Skills Scales
Performance Assessment of Self-Care Skills

Which assessments are used for Cognition?
Loewenstein Occupational Cognitive Assessment
Allen Cognitive Levels Screen
Cognitive Performance Test
Task Inventory
Diagnostic Modules

Dynamic Assessment of Categorization (Toglia Cognitive Assessment)

Which assessments are used for Work?
Jacobs Pre-vocational Assessment
Pre-vocational Screening
The Work Environment Impact Scale

Which assessments are used for Sensory Integration?
Schroeder-Block-Campbell
Touch Inventory for Elementary School Aged Children
Sensorimotor History (2 forms)
Sensory Integration Inventory-Revised
Sensory Profile—Original, Infant/Toddler, Adolescent/Adult

Which assessments are used for Projective?
Magazine Picture Collage
Kinetic Drawing System

Which assessments are used for Functional?
Kohlman Evaluation of Living Skills
Bay Area Functional Performance Evaluation
Independent Living Scales
Lowenstein Occupational Therapy Cognitive Assessment
Allen Cognitive Levels Screen
Cognitive Performance Test
Jacobs Pre-vocational Assessment
Schroeder-Block-Campbell

Which assessments are used for Social Interaction?
Assessment of Communication and Interaction Skills

Which assessments are used for Leisure?
Leisure Satisfaction Measure

What is the KELS method of assessment?
This test Combines interview & tasks.

What is the KELS population designed for?
For Low functioning populations.

What are the KELS 5 areas of living skills?
Self-care
Safety & Health
Money Management
Transportation & telephone
Work & Leisure

What is the problem with KELS assessment?
It relies on too much interview.

COPM (Canadian Occupational Performance Measure)

What is the method of data collection with COPM assessment?
Interviewing that is designed to Identify problems areas, evaluation performance, and measures change and the client's perception over time.

What is the population served by the COPM assessment?
All populations, with as variety of disabilities & developmental stages.

What areas are you assessing with the COPM?
Self-care
Productivity
Leisure

GENERAL OT

What is the method, what does it measure, and the population served by the SENSORY PROFILE assessment?
This is a checklist, subjective of style assessment that addresses sensory function

What does a COTA do to prepare to give an assessment?
Review or collect appropriate background and evaluation data
Decide if an assessment is appropriate. The OTR will determine, but with input from the OTA.
Create/locate an appropriate context for administering the assessment. (i.e. amount of furniture, hallway or classroom, etc.)
Communicate to the client the intent of the assessment and explain instructions.
Have the client complete the assessment.
Collaborate with the OTR on scoring, interpretation, and results.
Complete the planning and implementation plan for OT services, collaborative with OTR.
Review plan with client. Include client input. Depending on F.O.R. and assessment being used, the order of this will vary.

What are types of evaluations?
Interview
Functional
Structured Evaluations
Observation

What are the three levels of structure in evaluations?
Structured: you cannot deviate from the wording
Semi-structured: provides guidelines-may deviate from the wording given
Unstructured: no structure on how you perform it

What are examples of interview style assessments?
OPHI/OHI Occupational History Interview/Occupational Performance History Review
COPM Canadian Occupational Performance Measure
OCAIRS Occupational Circumstance Assessment Interview and Rating Scale Activity Configuration
TIE Touch Inventory of Elementary School Aged Children
Sensorimotor History
Sensory Integration Inventory-Revised
Routine Task Inventory
Prevocational Inventory

What are examples of functional style of assessments?

KELS
BAFPE
ILS
LOTCA
ACL
Cognitive Performance Test
Jacobs Prevocational Assessment
SBC
TCA

What is a structured evaluation?
Activities or series of activities following highly specific directions for administration and scoring, usually have norms, directions must be followed exactly

Define Assessments
Specific tests, instruments, interviews used to evaluate.

Define Evaluations
Planned process of collecting, interpreting and documenting information to plan intervention: overall process.

Define Service Competency
Mechanism to ensure that services are provided with the same high level of confidence
Defined as "the determination made by various methods, that two people performing the same or equivalent procedures will obtain the same or equivalent results – interpreter reliability

What does performing an evaluation tasks mean?
The ability of an occupational therapy assistant to obtain the same information as the supervising occupational therapist when evaluating a client's function.

Define Asset
Useful adaptive behavior used to help us get what is needed and carry out daily life activities.

Define Deficits
Behavior, which interferes with meeting needs.

What are the OTR/OTA roles in assessment?
OTR: Has overall responsibility

Choose method

Explains to the patient and family
Completes assessments
Organizes, analyzes and interprets information
Summarizes assets and deficits
Documents
Assigns roles to OTA
Establish service competency with OTA

OTA: Collects data as directed by OTR
With experience has more responsibility
Structured assessments
Organizes information and reports to OTR
Documents assessment
Collects information from record and observation and interviews
Establish service competency

The BAFPE is
Structured, functional and assesses ADLs.

Arthritis

What is Arthritis?
An inflammation of a joint or joints.

What are the types of arthritis?
Rheumatoid arthritis
osteoarthritis.

What is Rheumatoid arthritis?

Systemic, symmetrical and affects many joints.
Most commonly attacks the small joints of the hands.
Boutonniere and swan neck deformity are types of deformities.

What is Osteoarthritis?
Degenerative joint disease.
Not systemic, but wear and tear.
Commonly affects large weight bearing joints.

What is a Boutonniere deformity?
Flexion or PIP joint and hyperextension of DIP joint.

What is a Swan neck deformity?
Hyperextension of PIP joint and flexion of DIP joint.

Psychotropic Medications

What are MAOI's side effects and precautions?
Side effects: dietary restrictions, insomnia, and liver damage
Precautions: no food with AA tyramine (headache first sign, then increased blood pressure)

What are Mood stabilizing medication side effects and precautions?
Example: lithium
Side effects: excessive thirst, tremors, excessive urination, weight gain, nausea, diarrhea, and cognitive impairments
Precautions: monitor blood levels

What is a cyclothymic disorder?

It is a mood disorder characterized by a chronic pattern of relatively mild mood swings

What is dysthymia?
A low-grade chronic depression with symptoms that are milder than those of severe depression but are present on a majority of days for 2 or more years

What are the antipsychotic medications side effects?
Examples: mellaril, thorazine, prolixin, stelazine, trilafon, haldol, navane
Side effects: dry mouth, blurry vision, photosensitivity, constipation, orthostatic hypotension, akathisias, and tardive dyskinesia

What are Negative Schizophrenia symptoms?
Restricted emotion
Decreased thought and speech
Lack of motivation
Inability to relate to others

What is Fugue?
Individual takes on new identity

What are side effects to look for in Antianxiety medications?
Confusion

What are the side effects to look for in antipsychotic meds (neuroleptics)?
Akathisia
Extrapyramidal syndrome
Tardive dyskinesia.

Define Akathisia

Akathisia is a feeling of "inner restlessness", a constant urge to be moving.

It is peculiar in that while one cannot keep still, the actual movements are voluntary (as opposed to other movement disorders, such as tardive dyskinesia).

Anti-psychotic drugs often induce akathisia.

More rarely, it can be caused by anti-depressants.

What is the extrapyramidal syndrome?

Enables the person to engage more easily in activities in which physical coordination is a factor.

Abnormal movements, dry mouth, blurred vision, and nausea

Define Tardive dyskinesia.

Requires immediate medical intervention by doctor or nurse.

Involuntary movements of the face, trunk, and extremities.

Writhing motions of the tongue & fingers

Movement d/o that may become permanent unless patient stops taking the medication.

What do antipsychotic medicine help control?

Hallucinations and delusions and brings the person back into better contact with reality. To reduce violence in manic episodes and with drug abusers.

Requires frequent blood monitoring.

What were the negative symptoms of schizophrenia?

Apathy

Lack of interest in other people and one's environment, self-absorption, and lack of motivation.

What are Neuroleptics and Antipsychotic examples?
Chlorpromazine (thorazine)
Haldol

What is NMS?
Neuroleptic malignant syndrome.
Rare but life threatening effect of antipsychotic medications.
Signs: Extreme rigidity and Catatonia.
Any patient who suddenly becomes rigid or unresponsive
requires medical evaluation.

What is the therapeutic value of antidepressant drugs?
Relief from depression, suicide and social withdrawal.
Tricyclic's, MAOI's, SSRI's

What are the side effects of Tricyclic's?
Arrhythmia
Seizures
Urinary retention
Postural hypotension
Constipation.

What are the side effects of MAOI's?
Sweating
Palpations
Headache
Increases in blood pressure
TYRAMINE REACTION medical attention
Postural Hypotension
Vomiting and nausea
Drowsiness
Weakness

What are the side effects of SSRI's?
Sexual dysfunction
Anxiety
Insomnia
Nausea
Confusion
Agitation
Sweating
Shivering
Tremors
Jerky movements
Myoclonus
CENTRAL SEROTONIN SYNDROME requires immediate medical attention.

What should people taking MAOI's avoid?
Tyramine
Found in aged cheese, wine, beer, yogurt, tea, coffee, avocados, bananas, soy sauce, yeast, dates and raisins.

OT discipline and OTA/COTA info

What is a reprimand?
A private communication of disapproval of conduct.

What is censure?
Public disapproval statement (on NBCOT/AOTA) of a practitioner's conduct.

What is ineligibility?
Removal of eligibility of membership
Certification/licensure for a specific/indefinite time

What is probation?

A requirement for the individual to meet conditions (more education, more supervision, counseling, substance abuse training) in order to get license back.

What is suspension?

Loss of membership for a specific time

What is revocation?

Permanent loss of membership, certification, or licensure.

What roles can OTA/COTAs have?

Practitioners

Peer educations

Fieldwork educations

Administrators

Teachers

Entrepreneurs

What is the COTA/OTA's main role?

Implement treatment with orders from OTR

Cannot plan treatment by themselves

What does the COTA/OTA contribute to the evaluation process?

They can CONTRIBUTE to EVAL but cannot do it independently. They can do parts that do not require much tech skill, if the OTR determines this

OTA in SNF
Can be activity directors

Other OTA roles
Clerical, routine maintenance, prep for new session, CG during transfers.

Entry Level COTA Supervision and Supervises:
Close supervision by all levels of OTRs or advanced COTA under supervision of OTR. SUPERVISES: OT Aides, technicians, and care extenders, volunteers.

Intermediate COTA Supervision and Supervises:
Routine or general supervision by all levels or OTR's or advanced COTA under supervision of OTR.
SUPERVISES: Entry level COTA's, Level 1 OT fieldwork students, level 1 and 2 OTA fieldwork students.

Advanced COTA Supervision and Supervises:
General supervision by all levels of OTRs or advanced COTA under supervision of OTR. SUPERVISES: Intermediate COTA's.

MISC FACTS

What is a CHF level 1?
Not limited physical activity by pain, palpitations, angina, etc.

What is a CHF level 2?
Slightly limited physical activity, etc.

What is a CHF level 3?
Limited by physical activity, and during less than normal activity
Experiencing symptoms is common

What is a CHF level 4?
Unable to carry out physical activity without symptoms.
Symptoms at rest

What are behaviors and risks related to severe dementia?
Falls
Wandering
Safety
Hostile
Uncooperative

What is the cause of Carpel Tunnel?
Compression of median nerve- compressive neuropathy

What are Carpel Tunnel symptoms?
Numbness
Tingling in thumb and index
 Felt at night due to bending of wrists

When is the carpel tunnel onset?
After fracture
Secondary to medical condition
Continuous flexing

What is CRPS- complex regional pain syndrome?
Chronic pain following nerve injury
Affects extremities

What are CRPS symptoms?
Burning pain
Temperature changes on surface
Red/blotchy
Muscle atrophy
Less mobility

What is CRPS treatment?
ROM
Adaptive techniques
Work rehab,
Patient education
Nerve blocks
Medication
Psychotherapy
Surgery

Dyslexia is probably what kind of disorder?
neurological

What do patients with dyslexia have trouble relating to what?
Written word & letters
The sound they represent

What is pica?
An eating disorder in which patients eat non-food items

What diagnosis is pica generally seen with?
PDD

What is rumination disorder?
A disorder seen in infants in which they regurgitate and re-chew
food.
It is paired with arching back and sucking the tongue.

What causes rumination?
Neglect
Lack of stimulation

What is MD (muscular dystrophy)?
A gradual weakening of skeletal muscles

What is Duchenne MD?
Usually fatal before adulthood

What is Myotonic MD?
Muscle spasms
Heart
Endocrine problems
Drooping eyelids
Long thin face
Adult onset

What are MD child symptoms?
Enlarged, calf muscles
Gower's sign- standing with hands on front of legs due to weak
pelvic muscles

What does Parkinson's lead to?
Memory deficits
Dementia

What is done in Parkinson's treatment?
ROM
Strengthening
Balance/coordination
Retraining for ADLs
Energy conservation
Decrease risk of falls

OT HISTORY

Why is it important to study the history of OT?
The experience, social political, economic and religious influences. The changing ethic toward work.

Moral treatment
A change from prison like conditions to more humane treatment of people with mental illnesses. Age of Enlightenment.

Philippe Pinel
Father of Moral Treatment., a French physician who was instrumental in the development of a more humane psychological approach to the custody and care of psychiatric patients, referred to today as moral treatment. He also made notable contributions to the classification of mental disorders and has been described by some as "the father of modern psychiatry".

William Tuke
Society of Friends (Quakers) established the York Retreat.

Sir William and Lady Ellis
Regarded the hospital as a "community of family", established after care houses and night hospitals-these were half way houses to be used to help patients integrate into society easier.

Moral Treatment in the United Sates
Quakers brought ideas of moral treatment, by 1800's Dorthea Dix introduced the first patient bill of rights.

20th Century Progressivism
Not always so progressive. Industrial revolution led to increased work related injuries and chronic disabling disabilities.

Chicago's Hull House
Social experiment for immigrants and poor., Opened by Jane Addams in 1889 for immigrants to help with educational, social, and investigative programs.

Susan Tracey
The patient is the product not the article they make. Invalid occupations: keep the people busy, patient doing the process., Nurse credited for arts and crafts and for writing 1st known book for OTA "Studies invalid Occupations"

George Barton
Re-Education of Convalescents through employment, An architect with tuberculosis, nervous paralysis. Coined the term occupation. Founded the consolation house in Clifton Springs, N.Y.

William Dunton
Interest in the activity was paramount in his thinking. He had 9 principles to guide the emerging practice.1890-1920- another original founder of OT- editor of occupational therapy and rehabilitation - wrote numerous books about OT, Judious Regimen of Activity

Dorthea Dix
A women's rights activist that tried to improve public institutions. She used her grandparent's resources to set up charity schools to rescue abused children. She published 7

books, most imp was Conversations of Common Things. Was a treatise on natural science and moral improvement. Later she discovered insane women were jailed along side male criminals. She persuaded the Massachusetts lawmakers to enlarge the state hospital to accommodate mental patients. She began a national movement to establish separate, well-funded states hospitals for those with mental illnesses. She aroused public support.

Eleanor Clarke Slagle
Habit training,, MOTHER OF OT, credited with HABIT TRAINING, helped organize first professional OT school, her home was UNOFFICIAL headquarters for very first AOTA

Adolf Meyer
A Swiss physician who immigrated to the us in 1892 and later became a professor of psychiatry who expressed a point of view that eventually formed the philosophical base of profession of occupational therapy, holistic approach; he was committed to a holistic perspective and developed the psychobiological approach to mental illness, balance of habits, work, and leisure, -Involvement in meaningful activity

The founding of AOTA
The first title Society for the Promotion of Occupation Re-Education

The 1925 Principles
Purposeful work and leisure, involvement of mind and body, Occupational Therapy as a Learning Process, and the practioner's personal qualities.

Col. Ruth Robinson

President of AOTA military person, military wanted supportive personnel.

Marion Crampton
Massachusetts dept. of mental health, established one month in-service for OTA's

Mildred Schwagmeyer
AOTA director of technical education, training of OTA moved from hospital based to academic based. The most knowledgeable in the area of OTA's.

Ruth Brunyate Wiemer
President of AOTA, lead the OTA's through the changes taking place.

Individuals and Populations Receiving OT services
All age groups, all socioeconomic and cultural backgrounds, people with impairments, activity limitations, participation restrictions ,and any population that would benefit from health promotion.

Sites of intervention
Institutional settings, impatient hospitals, impatient mental health, impatient rehab, impatient mental health, sub-acute units/transitional care, nursing facilities, and prisons.

Outpatient Settings
Hospital, clinics, office visits, rehab, and partial hospitalization.

Home and Community Settings

Home care, halfway houses, group homes, assisted living, sheltered workshops, industry, business, schools, early intervention centers, day-care centers, community mental health centers, hospice, and wellness and fitness centers.

Occupational Performance Standards
Independence in ADL's, work and productive activities, play/leisure, and performance component function.

Quality of life
Purposeful participation as a member of a community, emotional well being, sleep and rest, energy and vitality, and life satisfaction.

Team members and the OT/OTA relationship
Intervention approaches, remediation/restoration, compensation/adaptation, disability prevention, and health promotion.

Why is it important for OT practitioners to have an understanding of, the philosophical base of the profession.
Provides an understanding of how the profession views the nature of existence, guides the actions of practitioners, as professionals, enables the profession to grow because it enables practitioners to explain reason for existence, it also ensures the survival of the profession. Explains why certain techniques are used and allows practitioners to communicate the value of these techniques to the patient.

What is metaphysics?
The ultimate nature of things, including the nature of man, the mind/body relationship, and holistic vs. dualistic. What is man?

Epistemology
The study of truth. Is concerned with the question of truth, how we know what we know, experience, intuition, feelings, and emotions.

Axiology
The study of values. Aesthetic component: What is beautiful in the world? ETHICAL- WHAT ARE THE RULES OF RIGHT CONDUCT

The evolution of OT
OT evolved from the moral treatment movement in the 19th century, it is based on Meyer's views about man, life, and a life worth living. This carried on into the 20th century.

The philosophy of Adolf Meyer
Carried his philosophies into the 20th century. What is man? Views man as holistic, man possesses a sense of time (past, present, and future) man has the capacity for imagination, and man has the need for occupation.

How does man know what he knows? EPISTIMOLOGY
Having the patient do rather than doing the patient.

What is beautiful or desirable in the world? AXIOLOGY ASTHETIC COMPONENT
Engaging the total self that man comes to experience the pleasure in achievements. Minimizing the deficits and maximizing the strengths.

What are the rules of right conduct? AXIOLOGY ETHICAL COMPONENT

Perceive patient not as an object, but as a person. Lacking the opportunity to do, man, like the squirrel, cannot control his destiny.

Current Philosophy of Occupation?

Man is an active being who participates in purposeful activity for life satisfaction. OT's use of purposeful activity and occupation can improve man's well being and health. Essential to providing OT services is a belief in our core values and attitudes. These include altruism, equality, freedom, justice, dignity, truth, and prudence.

Patient history

Each patient is unique, so each treatment approach must be individualized. Gather family information, vocational information, leisure and socialization.

Environmental Considerations

All conditions that influence and modify a person's lifestyle and activity level.

External environment

Climate-severe weather hazards or extreme temperatures, the effects of psyche, and effects on leisure activities.

Community

Urban, rural, suburban, effect on occupation, activities, and lifestyle.

Internal environment

Mood, emotional state, self-awareness, and self-image.

Economic environment
Effects on occupations, job availability, salary, insurance coverage, and equipment.

Sociocultural considerations
Ethic or religious groups that share belief or behaviors patterns. Matriarchal vs. Patriarchal cultures for example.

Customs
Holidays: 4th of July. Pattern or behavior that is common in a group, it is handed down form generation to generations.

Traditions
How you do the celebration, inherited patterns of thought or actions, surround certain occasions, i.e. birthdays and holidays.

Superstitions
Beliefs or practices resulting from ignorance or fear of the unknown.

Values, standards, and attitudes
Very personal and unique to the individual, may impact our intervention.

Severe disruptions
Sudden changes, usually superimposed-high stress.

Health
A state of complete physical, mental and social well-being. Not just an absence of disease.

Lifestyle Redesign
The key to lifestyle redesign is Individual redesign. Customizing a person's routines of daily living to maximize health.

Areas of health promotion in OT
ADA counseling, assisted living, community wellness programs, community redesign, ergonomics, home and private consultation, and spirituality and hope.

ADA
The Americans with Disabilities Act of 1990.

Ergonomics
Study of movement to accomplish tasks.

Roster of Honor
AOTA's national award for OTAs for leadership in OT.

What is the OT Domain of Practice?
It outlines the areas in which services are provided

What is the purpose of the framework?
It clear articulates OT's focus on daily activities
Discuses interventions that promote engagement to support participation in context
Gives practitioners a way to think about, talk about and apply occupations

What are the areas of occupation?

ADL
IADL
Work
Leisure
Social Participation
Rest & Sleep
Education
Play

What are ADLs?
Activities of daily living
Taking care of oneself

What are IADLs?
Activities that support daily live

What is work?
Employment or volunteer activities

What is leisure?
 Time not working, sleeping, doing self-cares

What are aspects of the Domain?
Areas of Occupation
Client Factors
Performance skills
Context and environment
Activities demands
Performance patterns

What are client factors?
Abilities, characteristics, beliefs

What are performance skills?
Observable, concrete, goal directed actions used in daily life

What are performance patterns?

Habits, routines, roles, rituals

What is the context and environment?
Context – cultural, personal, temporal
Environment – external physical and social environments

What are activities demands?
The amount of effort needed for an activity

What are performance skills?
Sensory perception skills
Motor and praxis skills
Emotional regulation skills
Cognitive skills
Communication skills
Social skills

What are habits?
Automatic behaviors

What are routines?
Patterns that are observable, regular and repetitive

What are rituals?
Symbolic actions with spiritual, cultural or social meaning

What does cultural refer to?
Expectations by the society a personal belongs to

What does personal refer to?
Age, gender, status, financial, education

FRAMEWORKS

Physical Function Frameworks

Biomechanical
originated by Bolderin, Taylor, and Licht

Neurodevelopmental Treatment
Originated by Berta ad Karl Bobath

Rehabilitation FOR
originated by Dunton

Proprioceptive Neuromuscular Facilitation
Originated by Kabat

Psychosocial Frameworks

Role Acquisition
Originated by Anne C Mosey

The Behavioral FOR
Adapted from Bruce & Borg

The Psychodynamic FOR
adapted from Bruce & Borg

PEDIATRIC-FOCUSED FOR

Motor Skills Acquisition
originated from Gentile
Sensory Integration
originated by Ayres

COGNITIVE/PERCEPTUAL FOR

cognitive rehabilitation
developed by OT's at Lowenstein Rehab Hospital

Dynamic Interactional
originated by Toglia

The Neuro-functional Approach
developed by Giles, Clark- Wilson, Yuen

MODELS USED IN OT

Client- centered models
Originated by Law, Christian, and Baum

Model of Human Occupation
originated by Reilly and Kielhofner

Occupational adaptation
originated by Schkade & Schultz

Occupational Science

originated by Yerxa

FIELD WORK

What are the three steps of acquiring a new skill?
1. Instruction
2. Practice
3. Patience

What requires the S and the O for reimbursement?
Medicare part B and managed care.

When was the OTPF developed?
2002

What does the OTPF stands for?
Occupational Therapy Practice Framework.

The OTPF is a useful resource for doing what?
documenting professional terminology.

What does SOAP stands for?
Subjective Objective Assessment Plan

How does the OTPF describe the domain of OT?
Engagement in occupation to support participation in context(s)

What are the three divisions of the occupational profile (OTPF)?

1. Influencing Contexts
2. Underlying Factors
3. Performance Skills

What is the purpose of the SOAP?
For documentation for and reimbursement from managed care and Medicare Part B.
To obtain preauthorization
Form of communication
It's a legal document.

What is a Problem Oriented Medical Record (POMR)?
SOAP notes.

When was the SOAP note developed and by whom?
1960's by Lawrence Weed.

What was the purpose for developing the POMR?
To make record keeping client centered.

What are the users and the uses of the health record (the first three only)?
1. Client care management. (multidisciplinary communication)
2. Reimbursement. (Medicare Plan B requires SOAP format)
3. Legal document.

What is the S (subjective) portion report?
To client's perception, subject perception

What is the O (objective) portion report?
The health professional's observations, objective perception

What are the 3 vital aspects of the O (objective) portion?
1. Measurable
2. Quantifiable
3. Observable

Only facility approved abbreviations are used. (T or F)
True.

What are the four things that should be indicated in the health record?
1. What services were provided, where and when.
2. What happened and what was said.
3. How the client responded to the service provided.
4. Why skilled OT services were needed (rather than those of an aide or a family member).

What are the mechanics of documentation?
1. Use waterproof black ink.
2. No correction fluid.
3. Do not erase.
4. No blank spaces.
5. Draw a line through errors then date and sign.

6. All data present.
7. Sign and date every note.
8. Be concise.
9. Appropriate terminology.
10. Prudence with abbreviations.
11. Refer to the clinician (yourself) in the 3rd person.
12. Spelling and grammar.
13. Notes continued write "(cont.)", on next page write date and "(OT note cont.)"
14. Adhere to ethical and legal guidelines.

15. Be honest and objective.
16. Write legibly.

What is the purpose of a Level 1 rotation, the community experience?
Exposure to different populations in different settings
To begin applying academic knowledge to real life situations.

Does a Level 1 rotation have to be supervised by an OT practitioner?
No. A Level 1 rotation can be supervised by non-OT personnel.

What is the purpose of a Level 2 rotation?
To prove competence in setting

Does a Level 2 rotation have to be supervised by an OT practitioner?
Yes, because skill competence is required

Define "skilled services".
Require professional education, complex competencies and decision making.

Define "non-skilled" services.
Routine or maintenance therapy.

What are the 3 reimbursable service categories?
1. Skilled services.
2. Safety concerns.
3. Prevention of secondary complications.

What are the 6 types of notes?
1. Initial evaluation reports.
2. Contact notes.
3. Progress notes.
4. Reevaluation notes.
5. Transition notes.
6. Discharge or discontinuation notes.

When writing a medical record what is the first thing that you write?
The introduction statement.

What are the 2 styles of writing the Observable portion of the medical record?
1. Chronological
2. Categorical

What are the 6 suggested categories for the O portion of the note from the OTPF?
1. Areas of Occupation
2. Performance skills
3. Performance patterns
4. Activity demands
5. Contexts
6. Client factors.

What must the introduction statement of the O portion include?
1. Length of Time
2. Where
3. For what reason

What is included in the second section of the O portion of the note?
Report observation, either chronologically or categorically.

What are the 6 reminders when writing the O portion of the note?
1. Deemphasize the media.
2. Specify what the part of the task the assistance was for.
3. Show skilled OT happening.
4. Leave yourself out.
5. Focus on the client's response.
6. Avoid being judgmental.

What is an ITP? What population is it used for?
Individualized.
Treatment.
Plan.
Birth-3 y/o with a focus on family, child and play as part of the IFSP.

What is an IEP? What is it for? What setting is it used in?
Individualized Education Plan.
For 3-18 y/o with a focus on education.
School setting

What is a DAP note? What are they? Where are they used?
Data Assessment Plan.
An adaptation from the SOAP notes, the D contains the S and the O.
A is clinicians interpretation.
Mental Health Settings. Skilled Nursing Facilities.

What is a BIRP note? What Population are they used with?
Behavior exhibited by the client

Intervention (is the O& some A)
Response to treatment (O)
Plan for continued treatment based on client's response (P)
Mental Health. (commonly used with Autism)

What is a PIRP note? (same as BIRP but for P)
Problems.
Interventions.
Response.
Plan.

What is an MDS note? What is its use? Where is it used?
Minimum Data Set.
To determine level of care by assessing all aspects of the patient.
Skilled nursing facilities.

What is a RUG note? What is it for? Where is it used?
Resource Utilization Groupings.
Determines reimbursement.
Skilled Nursing Facility.

What are the stages of and the notes taken during the intervention process?
1. Referral
2. Intake Note (who the client is, why OT referral, concerns and priorities, assessment results)
3. Intervention Plan (specific areas of occupation to be addressed)
4. Contact Note (each and every contact) (and/or)
5. Progress Note (at set intervals)
6. Reassessment Note (at regular intervals)
7. Transition Note
8. Discharges or Discontinuation Note

What is the focus of the intervention plan in a mental health setting.
Anger management
Stress management
Impact on ability to engage in occupation

What is documented in a Skilled Nursing Facility?
Function
Safety
Quality of life
Return home.

What is included in the subjective part of the SOAP note?
Client's report of limitations, concerns, problems, feelings, attitudes, concerns, goals & their plans.

What is a POMR?
This is the basis of the SOAP format.

Statements in the objective part of the SOAP note must be what?
Observable, measurable, quantifiable.

What are the two styles of objective reporting?
Chronological
Categorical organization.

What are the Performance Skills?
Cognitive
Motor& praxis
Sensory/perceptual

Communication
Emotional regulation

What are Client Factors?
Values and beliefs
Body structures
Body functions

What are the activity demands?
Space
Social
Cultural
Temporal
Physical
Virtual.

What are the 4 steps to writing a good O?
Begin with a statement about the setting and purpose of the activity.
Follow the opening sentence with a summary of what you observed.
Don't duplicate services.
Make your note professional, concise and specific.

8 questions to ask yourself when working on dressing:
1. What is the cognitive level of the child?
2. How does the child best learn?
3. Does a verbal explanation help or cause confusion?
4. Would a picture sequence help?
5. How much ROM and coordination are needed
6. Does the child perform symmetrical tasks?
7. What is the child's fine motor like?
8. Does the child have enough endurance to practice?

What are different types of dressing equipment for children?
Dressing Stick: long wooden shaft and plastic coated hooks on each end. One a "C" shaped hook and one "push-pull" hook.
Reacher: Aluminum shaft with a pulling lug (trigger) on one end and a clamp jaw on the other end.
Button hook: A hook or wire loop attached to a built up, rubber handle.
Zipper grip: Plastic grip with ring attaches to a zipper.
Shoe remover: Plastic shoe pedal sits on the floor for hands free removal of shoes.
Sock aid: Plastic material extended built up handle.
Elastic shoelaces: Coiled shoelaces eliminate the need for tying shoes.
Long handled shoehorn: Used to put on and take off shoes.
Dressing vest: Vest to practice snapping, buttoning, lacing, and zipping using oversized fasteners.
Tumble Forms: Used to help children with excessive or low tone to maintain a prone, seated or side lying position while performing ADLs, playing or resting.
Bow ties
Velcro shoe closure

What are adaptations for dressing?
Use oversized shirts and dresses
Choose pants and skirts with elastic waistbands
Sitting with back support while donning/doffing socks
Use footstool

What are activities that allow for dressing practice?
Fastening
 ~ Fastening boards or cubes
 ~ Play dress up
 ~ Dress up dolls

For Zipping
 ~ Oversized zipper
 ~ Zipping board

Abbreviations

'

feet

°

degree

1x/mo
once a month

1x/wk
once a week

2x/mo
twice a month

2x/wk
twice a week

3x/mo
three times a month

3x/wk
three times a week

AAOx3

alert, awake and oriented to person, place and time [times three]

AAROM
active assisted range of motion

ABG
arterial blood gasses

ACL
anterior cruciate ligament

ad lib
at liberty, as desired

ADA
Americans with Disabilities Act

ADD
attention deficit disorder

ADHD
attention deficit hyperactivity disorder

ADL
Activities of Daily Living (not ADLs or ADL's)

AE
above elbow

AFO
ankle-foot orthosis

AIDS
Acquired Immune Deficiency Syndrome

AKA
above knee amputation

ALS
amyotrophic lateral sclerosis

amb
ambulation; ambulates

ant
anterior

AP
advanced practitioner, for OTAs and COTAs only

AP
anterior-posterior

APE
adaptive physical education

APGAR
appearance, pulse, grimace, activity, respiration

AROM
active range of motion

ASHD
atherosclerotic heart disease

Ax
activity

BADL
Basic Activities of Daily Living

bid
twice a day

BKA

below knee amputation

BMI
body mass index

BP
blood pressure

CA (or ca)
cancer

CABG
coronary artery bypass graft

CAD
coronary artery disease

CARF
Commission on Accreditation of Rehabilitation Facilities

cath
catheter

CBI
closed brain injury

CBR
complete bed rest

CBT
cognitive behavioral therapy

CC (or C/C)
chief complaint

CCU
cardiac care unit

CDC
Centers for Disease Control and Prevention

CEU
Continuing Education Unit (10 contact hours)

CF
cystic fibrosis

CFS
chronic fatigue syndrome

CHF
congestive heart failure

CI
clinical instructor

CMS
Center for Medicare and Medicaid Services, formerly HCFA

CN
cranial nerve

CNS
central nervous system

COLD
chronic obstructive lung disease

cont.
continue

COPD
Chronic Obstructive Pulmonary Disease

CORF
certified outpatient rehabilitation facility

COTA
Certified Occupational Therapy Assistant

COTA/L
certified occupational therapy assistant, licensed

CP
cerebral palsy

CP
cold pack

CPM
continuous passive motion

CPMM
continuous passive motion machine

CPR
Cardiopulmonary Resuscitation

CPT
Current Procedural Terminology, a coding system used to bill for medical procedures

CQI
Continuous Quality Improvement

CSF
cerebrospinal fluid

CT
chest tube

CTR
carpal tunnel release

CTS
carpal tunnel syndrome

CVA
cerebral vascular accident

DC
doctor of chiropractic

DD
developmental disabilities, dual diagnosis

DDD
degenerative disc disease

DF
dorsiflexion

DHHS
Department of Health and Human Services

DIP
distal interphalangeal joint

DJD
degenerative joint disease

DM
diabetes mellitus

DME
durable medical equipment

DNR
do not resuscitate

DO
doctor of osteopathy

DOB
date of birth

DOE
dyspnea on exertion

DOE
Department of Education

DOL
Department of Labor

DRG
diagnostic-related group

DSM IV
Diagnostic and Statistical Manual of Mental Disorders - 4th
Edition

DT
delirium tremons

DTR
deep tendon reflex

DVT
deep vein thrombosis

Dx
diagnosis

EBV
Epstein Barr virus

ECG or EKG
electrocardiogram

EEG
electroencephalogram

EENT
ears, eyes, nose and throat

EI
early intervention

ER
emergency room

ETOH
alcohol [use or abuse]

ex
exercise

ext.
extension

F or f
fair

f/u
follow-up

FAOTA
Fellow of the American Occupational Therapy Association

FDA
Food and Drug Administration

FIM
functional independence measure

flex
flexion

Fx
fracture

Fx ROM
functional range of motion

G
good

G-tube
gastrostomy tube

GBS
Guillain-Barre Syndrome

GCS
Glasglow coma scale

GERD
gastroesophoageal reflux disease

GI
gastrointestinal

GYN
gynecologic

H&P
history and physical

HCFA
Health Care Financing Administration

hemi
hemiplegia

HHA

home health aide

HHA
Home health agency

HIPAA
Health Insurance Portability and Accountability Act

HIV
human immunodeficiency virus

HME
home medical equipment

HMO
Health Maintenance Organization

HOH
hard of hearing; hand over hand

HP
hot pack

HPI
history of present illness

HR
heart rate

Hx
history of

I&O
intake and output

IADL
Instrumental Activities of Daily Living

ICD-9
International Classification of Diseases, Ninth Edition

ICU
intensive care unit

IDDM
insulin-dependent diabetes mellitus

IDEA
Individuals with Disabilities Education Act

IEP
Individualized Education Program

IFSP
Individualized Family Service Plan

IM
intramuscular

IP
Interphalangeal

IRB
Institutional Review Board

JCAHO
Joint Commission on Accreditation of Health Organizations

JRA
juvenile rheumatoid arthritis

joint
joint

LBQC
large-based quad cane

LD
learning disability

LE
lower extremity -- leg

LLB
long leg brace

LLE (circled L)
left lower extremity

LOS
length of stay

LP
lumbar puncture

LPN
licensed practical nurse

LTC
long-term care

LTG
long-term goal

M O T
master of occupational therapy

MAOT
master of arts in occupational therapy

MCL
medical collateral ligament

MCP

Metatarsophalangeal

MD
medical doctor

MD
muscular dystrophy

MDS
Minimum Data Set

meds
medications; medicines

MHP
moist hot pack

ml
milliliter

mm
millimeter

mm-Hg
millimeters of mercury

MMSE
Mini-Mental Status Exams

mo.
month

MP
Metatarsophalangeal

MRI
magnetic resonance imaging

MRSA
methicillin resistant staphylococcus aureus

MS
multiple sclerosis

MSW
master of social work

MVA
motor vehicle accident

N
normal
or
normal, as in muscle grade

N/A
not applicable

NBCOT
National Board for Certification in Occupational Therapy

NDT
Neuro-Developmental Treatment

neg.
negative

NICU
neonatal intensive care unit

NIDDM
non-insulin-dependent diabetes mellitus

NIH
National Institutes of Health

NIOSH
National Institute for Occupational Safety and Health

NKA
no known allergies

NPO
nothing per mouth

NWB
non-weight bearing

O
objective

O2
oxygen

OA
osteoarthritis

OASIS
Outcome and Assessment Information Set

OBS
organic brain syndrome

OBS
observation

OCR
Office of Civil Rights (DHHS)

Oh
occupational history

OOB
out of bed

OP
outpatient

OR
operating room

OSHA
Occupational Safety and Health Administration

OT/s
occupational therapy student

OTA
occupational therapy assistant

OTA/L
licensed occupational therapy assistant

OTA/s
occupational therapy assistant student

OTC
over the counter

OTD
Doctor of OT (clinical doctorate)

OTR
Occupational Therapist Registered

OTR/L
occupational therapist, registered and licensed

P
plan; poor; pulse

PA

physician's assistant

PADL
Personal Activities of Daily Living

PAMS
physical agent modalities

para
paraplegic

PCA
personal care attendant

PDD
pervasive developmental disorder

Phys Dys
physical disabilities

PIP
Proximal Interphalangeal (Joint)

PLOF
previous level of function

PMH
past medical history

PMHx
past medical history

PNF
proprioceptive neuromuscular facilitation

PNI
peripheral nerve injury

PPO
Preferred Provider Organization

PPS
Prospective Payment System

PROM
passive range of motion

psych
psychology; psychiatry, psychiatric

PT
physical therapist

PTA
physical therapist assistant

PTA
prior to admission

PTS
Patient

PTSD
Posttraumatic stress disorder

PVD
peripheral vascular disease

PWB
partial weight bearing

Px
physical examination

q

every

QA
Quality Assurance

qd
once a day

QI
Quality Improvement

qid
four times a day

QM
Quality Management

QUAD or quad
quadriplegia; quadriplegic

r/o
rule out

RA
rheumatoid arthritis

RAS
reticular activating system

RD
registered dietician

rehab
rehabilitation

RN
registered nurse

ROH
Roster of Honor

ROM
range of motion

RROM
resisted range of motion

RUE (circled R)
right upper extremity

RUGS
Resource Utilization Groups

RW
rolling walker

Rx
therapy

S
subjective

S&S or S/S
signs and symptoms

SBA
stand by assist

SCI
spinal cord injury

SI
sensory integration

SIDS
sudden infant death syndrome

SLB
short leg brace

SLP
speech-language pathologist

SOAP
Subjective, Objective, Assessment, Plan Components of the Problem-Oriented Medical Record

SOB
shortness of breath

SSA
Social Security Administration

SSN
Social Security number

STD
sexually transmitted disease

STNR
symmetrical tonic neck reflex

sup
superior; supine

Sx
symptom

TB
tuberculosis

TBI
traumatic brain injury

TDD
telecommunications device for the deaf

TDWB
touch down weight bearing

TEDS
thrombo-embolic disease stockings

THA
total hip arthroplasty

ther ex
therapeutic exercise

THR
total hip replacement

TIA
transient ischemic attack

tid
three times a day

TKA
total knee arthroplasty

TKR
total knee replacement

TO or t.o.
telephone order

TPN
total parenteral nutrition

TQM
Total Quality Management

TS
tartive dyskinesia

TTWB
toe touch weight bearing

TTY/TDD
Teletypewriter/telecommunication device for the deaf

TWB
total weight bearing

Tx
treatment or traction

UE
upper extremity -- arm

UR
Utilization Review

UTI
urinary tract infection

v.s.
vital signs

VA
Veterans Administration

vent
ventilator

WHEELCHAIR or Wheelchair
wheelchair

WBAT

weight bearing as tolerated

WBQC
wide base quad cane

WFL
within function limits

WHO
World Health Organization

WNL
within normal limits

WP or wpl
whirlpool

$\bar{x}$
except for

X or x
Times

inches

↑ increased, up

↓ decreased, down

→ toward

←→ to and from

+ positive, plus

- negative, minus

= equal

~ approximately

Δ change

♀ female

♂ male

< less than

> greater than

✓ flexion

/ extension; per

c (with over line) with

p (with over line) post, after

s (with over line) without

Patient Safety Abbreviations

a
before

a.c.
before meals

A.M.

morning

A.S.A.
aspirin

abd
abdomen

ad lib
freely, as desired

adm
admission

AMA
Against Medical Advice

ASAP
As Soon As Possible

ASCVD
Arteriosclerotic Cardiovascular Disease

ASHD
Arteriosclerotic Heart Disease

B.M.
bowel movement

B.M.R.
basal metabolic rate

B.R.P.
bathroom privileges

B.U.N.
blood urea nitrogen

B/P
blood pressure

Ba E
barium enema

BPH
Benign Prostatic Hypertrophy

Bx
biopsy

c
with

C & B
chair and bed

C.

Centigrade, Celsius

C.B.C.
complete blood count

C.H.F.
congestive heart failure

C.O.P.D.
chronic obstructive pulmonary disease

C.V.A.
cerebral vascular accident

c/s or C & S
culture and sensitivity

Ca
Cancer or calcium

CABG
Coronary artery bypass graft

CAD
Coronary artery disease

cc
cubic centimeter

cl. liq.
clear liquids

CPR
cardiopulmonary resuscitation

CPT
chest physiotherapy

CVA
Cerebrovascular accident

CXR
chest x-ray

cysto
cystoscopy

D.A.T.
diet as tolerated

D.S.D.
dry sterile dressing

D.T.'s
delirium tremens

DM

Diabetes mellitus

DNR
Do Not Resuscitate

Dx
diagnosis

E.E.G.
electroencephalogram

E.E.N.T.
eyes, ears, nose and throat

E.K.G./E.C.G.
electrocardiogram

E.R.
emergency room

elix
elixir

Exc.
excision

F.
Fahrenheit

F.B.S.
fasting blood sugar

F.H.
fetal heart

F.Hx
family history

F.U.O.
fever of unknown origin

Fld.
fluid

G.B.
gall bladder

G.I.
gastrointestinal

G.T.T.
Glucose Tolerance Test

G.U.
Genital-urinary

gm./Gm.

gram

gtt.
Drop

H.C.V.D.
hypertensive cardiovascular disease

h.s.
hour of sleep

H/A
headache

h/o
history of

H2O
water

hct
hematocrit

hgb
hemoglobin

hgt.
height

HOB
head of Bed

HPI
History of present Illness

hs
Hour of sleep

HTN (BP)
Hypertension

Hx
history

I&D
Incision and Drainage

I&O
Intake and Output

I.M.
intramuscular

I.P.P.B.
Intermittent Positive Pressure Breathing

I.V.

intravenous

I.V.P.
intravenous pyelogram

KCl
potassium chloride

L
liter

L.L.L.
left lower lobe

L.L.Q.
left lower quadrant

L.P.
Lumbar Puncture

L.U.L.
left upper lobe

L.U.Q.
left upper quadrant

lb.
pound

liq.
liquid

M.O.M.
Milk of Magnesia

M.S.
Morphine Sulfate or Multiple Sclerosis

MAE
Move all extremities

mEq
mille-equivalent

mgm./mg.
milligram

MI
Myocardial Infarction (hear attack)

ml.
milliliter

N.P.O.
nothing by mouth

N/V

Nausea and vomiting

NAD
no apparent distress

Neg
negative

NG
nasogastric

NKA
No known allergies

NKDA
No known drug allergies

noc
night

NS
Normal saline

O&P
ova and parasites

O.D.
right eye

O.O.B.
out of bed

O.P.D.
Outpatient department

O.R.
Operating Room

O.S.
left eye

O.U.
both eyes

O2
oxygen

occ. bld., OB
occult blood

Ortho.
orthopedics

OT
Occupational therapy

p

after

P
pulse

p.c.
after meals

P.D. & P.T.
Postural drainage and (chest) physiotherapy

P.D.R.
Physician's Desk Reference

p.o.
by mouth

P.P.B.S.
post-prandial blood sugar (after meals)

P.P.D.
purified protein derivative

P.T.
Physical therapy

PE
Physical exam

Pedi.
Pediatrics

PERRLA
Pupils equal, round and reactive to light & accommodation

PMH
Past Medical History

post-op
Postoperative, after surgery

pre-op
Preoperative, before surgery

Prep
preparation

prn
as necessary

PVD
Peripheral vascular disease

Q 1o, 2o etc.
every 1hour, 2 hours etc.

q.s.

quantity sufficient

R
respirations

R.L.L.
right lower lobe

R.L.Q.
right lower quadrant

R.O.J.M.
range of joint motion

R.O.M.
range of motion

R.U.L.
right upper lobe

R.U.Q.
right upper quadrant

R/O
Rule out

ROS
Review of Systems

Rx
treatment/ therapy

s̄
without

S.C.
subcutaneous

S.G.
specific gravity

S.L.
sublingual

s.o.b.
short of breath

S.S., SOS
Sacraments of the Sick

S.S.E.
soap suds enema

S.T.D.
Sexually Transmitted Disease

s/p

Status post (status after)

s/s
signs and symptoms

sol.
solution

Stat, STAT
immediately

Sx
symptoms

syr.
syrup

T
Temperature

T.W.E.
tap water enema

tab.
tablet

TF
Tube feeding

tinct.
tincture

TPR
temperature, pulse, respiration

trans.
transfer

Tx
Traction, treatment

U.R.I.
Upper Respiratory Infection

U.T.I.
Urinary Tract Infection

u/a
urinalysis

ung.
ointment

v.s., VS
vital signs

W.B.C.

white blood count

WD
Well developed

WF
white female

WM
white male

WN
well nourished

WNL
within normal limits

wt./wgt.
weight

Development Editor: Stacy Hoffman
Technical Editors: Stacy Hoffman and Tim Hetfield
Production Editor: Colton McGovney
Copy Editor: Kristin Kenney
Editorial Manager: Larry Adams
Book Designers: Kori Callahan and Colton McGovney
Proofreader: 3 Point Farms Documentation, Inc.
Project Coordinator: River Kelly
Cover Designer: Colton McGovney

Exam Facts

CPSIA information can be obtained at www.ICGtesting.com
Printed in the USA
LVOW09s1656190813

348622LV00006B/977/P